The Life and Deaths
of Cyril Wecht

T0130743

The Life and Deaths of Cyril Wecht

Memoirs of America's Most
Controversial Forensic Pathologist

CYRIL H. WECHT, M.D., J.D.
and JEFF SEWALD

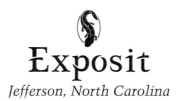

Exposit

Jefferson, North Carolina

Library of Congress Cataloguing-in-Publication Data

Names: Wecht, Cyril H., 1931– author. | Sewald, Jeffrey M., author.
Title: The life and deaths of Cyril Wecht : memoirs of America's most
controversial forensic pathologist / Cyril H. Wecht, M.D. and
Jeffrey M. Sewald.
Description: Jefferson, North Carolina : Exposit, 2020 | Includes index.
Identifiers: LCCN 2020022631 | ISBN 9781476684246
(paperback : acid free paper) ∞
ISBN 9781476642185 (ebook) ∞
Subjects: LCSH: Wecht, Cyril H., 1931- | Forensic pathologists—
United States—Biography. | Forensic pathology—United States—
Biography. | Forensic sciences—United States.
Classification: LCC RA1025.W43 A34 2020 | DDC 614/.1092 [B]—dc23
LC record available at https://lccn.loc.gov/2020022631

British Library cataloguing data are available

ISBN (print) 978-1-4766-8424-6
ISBN (ebook) 978-1-4766-4218-5

———

Front cover: Allegheny County Coroner Dr. Cyril Wecht
talks to the media regarding an inquest into the death
of Capus Jones, who died after a fight with a tow-truck driver.
June 28, 2001 (*Pittsburgh Post-Gazette*/Matt Freed).

Back cover: Former Allegheny County Coroner
turned celebrity pathologist Dr. Cyril Wecht
leaves the Federal courthouse in Pittsburgh.
January 28, 2008 (*AP* Photo/Don Wright).

Printed in the United States of America

Exposit is an imprint of McFarland & Company, Inc., Publishers

Exposit
Box 611, Jefferson, North Carolina 28640
www.expositbooks.com

This book is dedicated to my wife, Sigrid, whose love and devotion for almost six decades have provided the support and courage that have enabled me to survive the trials of an active and multifaceted career, and to have achieved some measure of success throughout difficult and turbulent times…

…and to my children, David and Valerie, Daniel and Anna, Benjamin and Flynne, Ingrid and Harold, and my 11 grandchildren, without whom all of the excitement, challenges, and feelings of accomplishment in my various professional and political endeavors would not have had the same significance and personal satisfaction.—C.H.W.

*"Cyril couldn't be intimidated if you faced him
with a Sherman tank."*

—F. Lee Bailey

Acknowledgments

I want to express my heartfelt gratitude to all the wonderful individuals whose candid historical reflections and gracious personal commentaries have provided an essential and meaningful component to this memoir. To all my academic and professional colleagues, former political allies and loyal supporters, and longtime personal friends, who generously provided their time to share their thoughts and experiences related to my activities throughout a 60-year career, I shall remain forever grateful.

My wife, Sigrid Wecht, Esq., and my children, Pennsylvania Supreme Court Justice David N. Wecht, Dr. Daniel A. Wecht, neurosurgeon, Benjamin E. Wecht, Director of the Cyril H. Wecht Institute of Forensic Science and Law, and Dr. Ingrid A. Wecht, obstetrician-gynecologist, provided consistent support and perceptive advice throughout the creation of this book.

Florence Johnson, my longtime secretary, and Joseph Mancuso, my dependable pathology assistant for almost fifty years, have also been very helpful in many ways.

This book would never have come to fruition without several years of intensive input of time and energy, personal dedication, keen perception, and journalistic ability by my coauthor, Jeff Sewald. His amiable personality and investigative skill enabled him to meet and talk with extremely busy, prominent people throughout the country to obtain the private comments that have made this volume meaningful, interesting and informative. Thank you, Jeff. I have truly enjoyed collaborating with you and developing a close friendship through this special endeavor.—C.H.W.

Table of Contents

Preface

This book depicts, in a condensed fashion, the major events of my life and career. It was not written as a commercial venture to attract more consultations to my business, or because I plan to run for political office again, or because I want to be more famous. I'm now 89 years old and my consulting schedule is still jammed, my days of running for office are behind me, and I'm already famous enough.

If it was just a matter of writing a book about my life for the general public, I might have considered doing it but, believe it or not, I don't feel the need to tell the world more about myself than they may already know. When it comes right down to it, I wrote this book, first and foremost, for my children and grandchildren, and those in my family who will come later. I want my family and, indeed, my close friends and loyal colleagues, to know my story as I see it.

In addition to summarizing the highlights of my life and work, this book also tells a darker, more cautionary tale resulting from instances of profound adversity, specifically two major legal actions that were brought against me for malevolent personal and political reasons. I'm proud to say that I prevailed in both instances but, in these pages, I've endeavored to memorialize and make clear the facts of those court cases. I want readers to understand that serious injustices do take place in this country. When individuals dare to stand up to the authorities, whether it's a local DA, a U.S. Attorney, or an agent of the FBI. These people, if sufficiently provoked, with support from their taxpayer-funded institutions, can and will set out to get you.

I've always believed that if I described the egregious nature of what some powerful people tried to do to me, and if I provided an overview of the battles I waged and the victories I ultimately achieved, others who find themselves in similar circumstances might come to believe that, if necessary, they, too, could take on the authorities, and win. Doing so, however, requires a great deal of courage and stamina, not to mention a supportive family, and strong, tough, competent attorneys. If you are truly not guilty of allegations made against you, and you are prepared to withstand tremendous pressure, I say, dig in and fight back.

Would these particular adversities have come about if I hadn't stayed in Pittsburgh my whole life? It's hard to say. Pittsburgh is a friendly place. It also can be rather provincial. My coauthor, Jeff Sewald, once told me that one of the things he likes most about me is that I seem to be loved and hated by all the right people, and there may be some truth in that. Contrary to the opinions of some, however, I don't go looking for trouble. But by way of my work in forensic pathology and legal medicine, and my longtime involvement in politics, I have often encountered situations about which I feel a responsibility to speak out, sometimes intensely. This propensity has made me the target of not only the derision of some loftily placed individuals, but also of certain institutions that do not want the truth to be told about them or their activities. When I express myself and take strong stands on particular issues, people lash out at me, and I don't back off.

Admittedly, sometimes I react too quickly. Perhaps I should take more time and think things through a little better. And I probably should be, not ameliorative or conciliatory, but maybe a bit less sensitive when it comes to disagreements. Had I been, in some instances, more patient or diplomatic, perhaps I might have achieved more in my life. But I'm proud of the fact that, even with my big mouth, and after all the controversial stands I've taken through the years, I still enjoy a great degree of acceptance, admiration and respect, at home and elsewhere.

All told, as a coroner and private consultant, I've probably done more exhumation autopsies than any other forensic pathologist in the country, because my work has involved me in many medical-legal matters. I once examined the remains of a person who had been buried for more than a century, and several who had been dead for twenty, thirty or forty years. Usually, however, I examine the remains of people who have been dead for much shorter periods of time. And after nearly sixty years and more than 100 exhumation autopsies, I still sometimes think, "What the hell is this?"

My nose is yours and my eyes are yours. I can smell and see what you smell and see. One can't be trained not to smell or not to see, and there are things to which one can't acclimatize. But it's the work that I do. For me, the most important thing is never to lose cognizance of the fact that I'm dealing with deceased *human beings*. Somebody, somewhere, at some time, loved these people. So, such situations must always be handled with dignity and respect. Those of us in forensic pathology recognize that what we do is very sensitive, and also extremely important.

In my work, I have examined many horrible things that have happened to everyday people in everyday life: murders, childhood deaths, tragic accidents and police brutality, to name some, and it is a wonder that I do not suffer from a malignant cynicism because of this. Admittedly, and I state this without hesitation and with a certain degree of pride, I feel passionate about the cases that come before me. I don't deal with any of them in a superficial fashion. And I reject statements made by anyone who believes that such matters, in the scheme of national and world events, are not all that important. How could I not be passionate about what I believe? It doesn't diminish or deprive me in any way to feel and react strongly about these "smaller" things. Show me a person who doesn't get excited about "small" things, and I'll show you a person who probably doesn't get too excited about "big" things either.

Sometimes comments come back to me, often snide, about my involvement in high-profile cases. Well, that's also what I do, as a well-known forensic pathologist. But my work on such cases hasn't kept me from consulting in hundreds of lower-profile civil and criminal cases every year, nor has it prevented me from doing the necessary autopsies. There aren't many pathologists around who have done more of them than me, and there aren't many who, at my age, are still doing them—more than 500 per year, on average.

At age 89, I still work seven days a week, and many evenings, too. I give interviews, in person and via telephone, even while I'm in the car. I get many requests from students, probably more than 100 over the years, who express an interest in forensic pathology and are writing papers or working on projects about some aspect of it, and I'll often ask them to call me at home when I'll have more time to spend with them. I speak quite often at high schools, colleges and universities, and at various community organizations, as well as at several national and international conferences conducted by medical-legal and forensic science professional organizations. If a person has that kind of work ethic, is a multi-tasker, and functions with great intensity, as I do, it's amazing how much can be accomplished.

In spite of my schedule, my wife, Sigrid, our four children, their spouses, and our 11 grandchildren, have managed to travel together for wonderful prolonged visits to, among other destinations, my wife's native Norway, and my cultural home, Israel. I have also lectured on cruise ships for many years, and have taken Sigrid and one of our children's families on each, whenever our grandkids' school schedules permitted. In fact, I'll bet we've spent more time with each other at home and elsewhere than most families. In the end, I believe that one does what one must, as determined by the internal compass of one's being—what the mind and heart require.—C.H.W.

"You shall judge a man by his enemies
as well as by his friends."
—Joseph Conrad

Introduction

Cyril Wecht grew up as the bright and only child of hard-working Jewish immigrants, shopkeepers who believed that, if he applied himself, he could grow up to be anything he wanted to be.

Born on March 20, 1931, in Bobtown, Pennsylvania, and raised in Pittsburgh, Cyril experienced a youth full of love, learning and activity. He helped at his family's grocery store. He excelled in school, endured intensive violin lessons, and participated in a host of sports. Like so many people who hailed from blue-collar families during the years of World War II, Cyril knew that success in America would come only as a result of personal effort and tenacity. He had no cushion, no inheritance on which to rely, and thus he became driven, passionate and ceaselessly active, desirous of any and all knowledge and experience at once. And while his life's course would twist and turn, and his fortunes rise and fall, the man's belief in himself never wavered. Cyril Wecht's life has been a testament to the resiliency of the human spirit.

Pittsburgh, in Cyril's time, was not always the ideal place for the most bold and progressive. By and large, its citizens were a conservative lot (despite their historical propensity to vote for Democrats). Having witnessed the shattering of their once-fabled image as makers of the "steel that built America," Pittsburghers have been forced to wrestle with the concept of just who and what they are now. Many take only the most calculated of chances. Many welcome outsiders, but cautiously. And many don't believe in rocking the boat.

Nonetheless, today the city remains a friendly place, resolutely on a path of evolution from industrial might to technological innovation. Blessed with charming neighborhoods and modern public amenities, Pittsburgh is, essentially, a great mid-sized Midwestern town with some skyscrapers, some exceptional universities and hospitals, and famous football and baseball franchises. It has its benefits, and its liabilities. But like many American towns these days, Pittsburgh sometimes fails to acknowledge the contributions it has made to its own setbacks, among which are manifestations of prejudice and racism. These have precipitated an uneasy relationship between local minorities and the city's government and police force. Cyril Wecht knows this. As a child of the once racially mixed Lower Hill District, he has fought throughout his professional life on issues of social and criminal justice. And it has often cost him, dearly.

Given the fascination that America has for true crime stories, this project to me was a natural. Time has proven that the public maintains strong feelings about and interest in many of the cases on which Cyril has worked for the past six decades as one of the nation's most celebrated forensic science experts. The public wants to lynch this perpetrator or that one, whether it's Lee Harvey Oswald, Claus von Bülow, O.J. Simpson, or Scott Peterson. These and other "villains" have become part of America's collective nightmare—a never-ending, reality-based Halloween replete with monsters of all shapes, sizes and persuasions.

Thirty years ago, true crime was but a small tract on the American publishing landscape. Back then, Vincent Bugliosi's *Helter Skelter*—about the investigation, trial and conviction of cult leader and mass-murderer Charles Manson and several of his followers—was a literary sensation that led, over time, to the rise of a multitude of ultra-successful true crime authors, and the eventual launching of cable television outlets such as *Court TV* (now *truTV*) and *Investigation Discovery*, both of which devote virtually their entire programming schedules to sensationalizing the misdeeds of an endless stream of miscreants and madmen.

The public's insatiable appetite for "ripped from the headlines" entertainment—which has, at its core, the horrors and tragedies of real human beings—is a peculiar phenomenon. But equally popular (and perhaps more socially palatable) is the crime scene investigation, or "CSI," strand of network television dramas that has dominated primetime television, and the AC Nielsen ratings—for many years now. Blame it on Universal Studios because the trend actually began as far back as 1976 with the formulaic but highly successful television series "Quincy, M.E.," which starred Jack Klugman in the title role as a strong-willed and principled Los Angeles County medical examiner. In truth, Cyril Wecht was "Quincy" way before Jack Klugman, *sans* the houseboat, of course, and *sans* the freedom to mercilessly browbeat the accused without allowing due process.

At an age when many American men have either already left us or are spending their time playing golf or sunning themselves in Florida, in 2008, Cyril found himself confronting a ginned-up, 84-count federal indictment for "abuse of public office." The trial that followed had an undercurrent of local political skullduggery and a gallery of colorful supporting players, including a hard-nosed defense attorney; a kindly Catholic nun who described the government agents who were seated in the courtroom during the trial as "a pack of mad dogs"; Mephistophelian federal prosecutors; a discredited FBI agent; and a conniving and soulless district attorney. Had our protagonist been caught in the vast and sticky web of dirty politics, professional opportunism, and personal revenge? We'll present Cyril's case.

In approaching Cyril Wecht and his life's story, I began not with the legend but with the man himself. Stepping into his Pittsburgh office to interview him for a magazine feature that I had been commissioned to write, I expected to encounter the intense, blustering and seemingly angry person that had often been depicted on the local evening news. To me, at the time, Cyril was just another local public official who had faced down rather sensational corruption charges. Like my regional brethren, I had been twisted by the media's somewhat simplistic portrayal of this indefatigable and loquacious county coroner and political player. The man I found instead was a lucid, self-aware, amazingly sharp and courteous, overworked gentleman in his eighties, who had suffered the slings and arrows of bloodless political opponents and other detractors for decades, and who definitely had a desire to tell his side of his story. For me, the prospects were irresistible.

Before I sought interviews with Cyril Wecht's many and impressive colleagues and friends, I spent more than 40 hours collecting the thoughts of the man himself, tracing his history and covering the highlights of his career, in and out of the spotlight. It wasn't until around hour number 15 that I witnessed Cyril sigh, look down at the floor, and begin to tell me not what he thought, but rather what he felt. It was only at that point that I knew we had a book in the making.

In the end, Cyril said, if we could memorialize in writing the importance of his profession and the highlights of his storied career, alongside the egregious personal and legal actions taken against him by powerful adversaries, as well as the facts surrounding his two courageous battles to vindicate himself, his life's story could prove meaningful and inspirational beyond the field of forensic science, and beyond the details of the many sensational cases in which he has played a part. "Everyone in America needs to know," Cyril told me, "that one really can beat those bastards," meaning the rogues that often abuse the authority of federal and state governments. He fought them, and beat them, and lived to tell about it.—J.S.

My Hometown

I was born in Bobtown, Greene County, near the West Virginia border, and was raised in Greater Pittsburgh, the latter of which was the final resting place of my parents and the birthplace of my children and grandchildren. The city has afforded me great opportunity, first as a student, then as a scientist, and even as a politician. I've made good friends and developed strong professional relationships here. I have praised all that is good about my hometown, and have courted controversy when I thought it had fallen short of being all that it could be.

SIGRID WECHT: *Cyril grew up in the Lower Hill District and went to Fifth Avenue High School, where the student body was very mixed. Through the years, he has often been disappointed with some things that have happened in Pittsburgh between the white population and minorities, especially African Americans. I think that, when you belong to a minority in this country—if you're Jewish like Cyril, or if you are black—you must have an urge not only to improve yourself, but to prove yourself, too. If you don't, life will likely be very difficult.*

Everyone knows that Jews have been persecuted throughout the centuries and maybe, somehow, those injustices live inside me. I became aware of this as a teenager, and even more so as a young man. It is correct to say that my lifelong feelings as a Jew, and my strong resentment of anti–Semitism, from verbal insults to the Holocaust, made me willing to fight, if necessary. How else can you explain why I behave the way I do when I'm provoked? Having my dukes up is just part of my personality.

When I was young, more than a dozen synagogues were located in Pittsburgh because of the various Polish, German, Lithuanian, Romanian and other Jewish populations that lived in the city. Each Jewish immigrant group wanted their own place of worship, and where you came from was the determining factor as to which synagogue you frequented. Nowadays, we have fewer but bigger synagogues, and the one at which you worship is determined by whether you are "Reform," "Conservative" or "Orthodox."

Over time, different sociological factors came into play to break down some of the barriers between people in Pittsburgh. And more than anything else, economics was at the core. Were you rich, middle-class or poor? One's place was determined more by what one earned than by who he or she was. Jews didn't move to ritzy Fox Chapel or Sewickley Heights back then, not because people weren't willing to sell to them, but

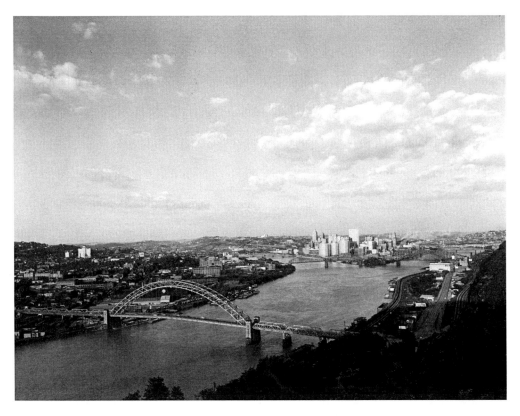

Pittsburgh in the early 1960s, where and when my long and winding career began (Carnegie Library of Pittsburgh).

because not many Jews had money enough to buy homes in those communities. But in time, we earned and then, of course, we moved.

Most people don't know that I served in the U.S. Air Force, but during my second year of service, I took leave to travel to Israel where I met up with my mother and my friend Dr. Arthur Grossman. Early on, I contacted my Congressman, William S. Moorhead, with whom I had become friendly, having campaigned for him before going into the service. Congressman Moorhead graciously provided me with tickets to attend one day of the trial of Nazi Adolf Eichmann. As a Jew, it seemed like my duty to observe while justice was done.

So, I went to the Eichmann trial, and there he was, seated in a glass case. I didn't get to hear him testify, but I did hear the testimony of Pennsylvania Supreme Court Justice Michael Musmanno. In that one day, I learned how a legal case was presented and how justice was served. And I was very impressed by the fact that the Israelis had given even the worst of men his day in court.

To this day, and maybe even more so with each passing year, I think about the Holocaust and what the Nazis did. I have very intense feelings about it, and am enraged by the fact that the Jews of Europe didn't fight but, rather, went like lambs to the slaughter. Of course, I wasn't there. And the Jews had no army. For a while, many of them didn't realize the extent of what was going on, or that many of their non–Jewish neighbors were willingly collaborating with the Germans to turn them in. But the question that most puzzles me is this: At what point does one, as a Jew, come to realize, for the safety of one's children if not for oneself, that the Nazis meant business? At what point does one say, "We must get the hell out of here." I am critical of those Jews who did not think first about their families. I might have angrily told the Nazi stormtroopers, "Go fuck yourselves," but not at the expense of my spouse, children or grandchildren.

RABBI ALVIN BERKUN: *Cyril is a person of strong opinions, and I can appreciate his perspective. Unfortunately, he hasn't always had the support of the Jewish community in Pittsburgh. On the other hand, I've rarely encountered anyone who has been more supportive of the State of Israel than Cyril, its existence and its positions. I came to Pittsburgh in 1983 and, by that time, Cyril had had some legal complications in his life that were troubling to the Jewish community. The Jewish establishment did seem to want him to go away, worried that he might bring shame. He certainly brought notoriety, because Cyril is not a "shrinking Jew." Most of the Jewish people I know admire him tremendously but still, there are those who don't.*

I'll admit that my personality has been a factor in some of my problems with the Jewish establishment because there are some Jews who prefer to dance between the raindrops. "Times are good. Why should we rock the boat?" For some reason, my unwillingness to tolerate bullshit or to accept deceitfulness and disingenuousness seems to bother these people. I may seem "pugnacious" at times, as some have described me, but not to the point of being arbitrarily or unnecessarily contentious. Others have labeled me "arrogant." But I contend that they simply misconstrue candor or forthrightness for arrogance. A person in Pittsburgh is deemed arrogant when he won't bend and go along. I don't consider myself difficult, except about things that matter.

DANIEL WECHT: *People generally love my dad, and I think love for my dad gets more pronounced as you go down the income scale. The more a person is focused on how much money they can make, the less my dad is going to be enamored of them.*

RABBI ALVIN BERKUN: *Cyril is extraordinarily bright, but more important than that is the commitment he has shown to the causes he holds dear. When I speak outside the Jewish community, I often find myself talking about his involvement with the African American community and police issues, and how he's come to the rescue of black people many times. To me, that's a sign of great character. He's been able to hold those positions and not be meek. To his credit, he's been out there fighting, sometimes alone. He has risen to the defense of people when there was nothing in it for him but grief, yet he did so because it was the right thing to do.*

WILLIAM ROBINSON: *I've probably known Cyril for 50 years, and I have a very good friend by the name of Louis Kendrick, we call him "Hop," who went to high school with him. Whenever we'd talk about black and white relations, he'd bring up Cyril's name. Cyril is someone in whom I have confidence. He is tenacious and straightforward. He's taken on some tough issues in this county for which he's paid a terrible price.*

BEV SMITH: *I don't know whether it's because of Cyril's ethnicity, being Jewish, that he can understand what it's like to be discriminated against. But he's experienced anti–Semitism and knows what it's like. I think he has a deep understanding that racism is deeply entrenched in Pittsburgh, but it's the kind of racism where people don't even know that they're racist.*

Growing up in the Lower Hill, I remember how some people behaved toward African Americans, especially the police. Detectives often coerced confessions from black suspects by dunking their heads in toilets and flushing. You may not want to believe it, but these things happened, right here in Allegheny County.

To keep things in perspective, let's consider the post–World War I period. "Jim Crow" was being played out in the South, the Ku Klux Klan was on the rise, and blacks were being oppressed and denied basic civil and, in some cases, human rights. Don't you think that there was more violence by police officers toward blacks then than there is now? You bet your ass there was. Perhaps life has become a bit more "civilized" over time because the average person is no longer willing to tolerate misbehavior by the police. My belief is that a segment of the police force has always been racist and abusive, and I'm pleased that it's now being uncovered.

> SALA UDIN: *In the late 1960s, police brutality was always the number-one civil rights issue in the community, or at least close to the top. When Cyril calls an instance of extreme police brutality toward a black person "homicide," he is seen as a friend of the black community, someone who stands up against cops, the DA, and judges who would turn a blind eye. Cyril has a history of taking on the system on behalf of justice in the eyes of many black people.*

> CHARLES MORRISON: *Some law enforcement officials are looking for someone to back up what they believe and think Dr. Wecht should go along. And many, unfortunately, are used to getting their way. They're hard-set that an incident had to have happened in a particular way. Some hard feelings have developed between law enforcement and Dr. Wecht because he lets the body speak for the scene and the evidence speak for the incident. And he is not shy. Based on his findings, sometimes he'll say to law enforcement, "You're absolutely wrong. This is the way it happened." All things considered, I don't think Dr. Wecht hates law enforcement. I don't think he personally picks fights with police officers. He speaks the truth of the evidence, and I trust his judgment. Thank God, most jurors do, too. I have nothing but good things to say about him.*

For 20 years, when I was Coroner of Allegheny County, I made sure that every police-related death was followed by a public "open inquest," presided over by a retired judge or, at least, several prominent members of the American Bar Association. But since I left office, the county Medical Examiner has stopped doing such inquests. Upset, I wrote a memo to the local news media asking what their feelings were about this. I got no response.

Normally, the media are all over me, looking for a story or at least some colorful quotes to splash across their pages or to inject into their broadcasts. Yet, when it comes to cases of significance involving the local police, which are rife with sociopolitical controversy and of great public importance, the media has been mostly silent. It doesn't bother them that the Allegheny County District Attorney alone gets to decide whether any charges can or will be brought against police officers who have been deemed purveyors of misdeeds. I'm not suggesting that police brutality is never recognized locally, but there isn't a hell of a lot being done about it.

JOHN MCINTIRE: *The establishment in this town does nothing but support the cops, and Cyril is definitely for the "little guy" when it comes to abuse of the public at the hands of police officers. Some might say that making enemies of the police is not a wise thing to do, but Cyril is fearless.*

Not long ago, before "Black Lives Matter," when it concerned black people, no one really gave a shit about police brutality. The public would get riled up by it temporarily, but would never follow through. I can't go so far as to suggest that a quasi-organized movement among police officers exists and allows these things to happen. That kind of conspiracy would be difficult to maintain. But the police don't need a cabal. They don't have to have a leadership that orchestrates nefarious and violent actions. I think that police brutality has persisted through the decades due to the low-level of knowledge and interest in government as demonstrated by the "fat and happy" American public and, dare I say it, racism.

Lessons in Malevolence

As the elected Coroner of Allegheny County—from 1970 to 1980, and again from 1996 to 2006—I built one of the most respected medical-legal investigative offices in the nation, and I also became an outspoken consultant on deaths with a high media profile. My expertise was utilized in the cases of John F. Kennedy, Robert F. Kennedy, Elvis Presley, Nicole Brown Simpson, JonBenét Ramsey and Laci Peterson, among many others. I also created unique forensic-science academic programs at Pittsburgh's Carlow and Duquesne universities. Even more, as Coroner, I established a high level of credibility and community acceptance of official findings that I issued in difficult and often controversial cases. Among these were police-related deaths, which are never easy to handle, for any coroner, in any jurisdiction.

In 1997, Bob Colville stepped down as Allegheny County DA after being elected to a judgeship on the Court of Common Pleas. His replacement, via appointment by the Common Pleas judges, was Stephen A. Zappala, Jr., a member of a prominent local family with strong political connections.

Zappala is the son of Stephen Zappala, Sr., who was a Justice, and later Chief Justice. of the Pennsylvania Supreme Court. Young Steve Zappala was a neophyte attorney with essentially no criminal law experience and little, if any, trial experience. But we soon learned that he would do his best to faithfully uphold Pittsburgh's law-enforcement tradition, especially when it came to African American suspects.

TIM UHRICH: *Anything and everything that Steve has ever achieved was by way of appointment. It's an old-time Pittsburgh thing: from fathers to sons; familial legacies. That's the way it has been here. But at the time, no one realized the true depths of Steve's megalomania.*

JOE DOMINICK: *I met Cyril when he returned to the Allegheny County Coroner's Office for the second time, in 1996. I had been working there as an investigator, mostly on the night shift, under the administration of Dr. Joshua Perper and, for a short time, Dr. Sanford Edberg. Eventually, I was promoted to a supervisory position, and worked in several capacities as a supervisor. Then, ultimately, when Jim Bentz, who was Chief Deputy Coroner, became ill, I became the Acting Chief Deputy. After Jim's death, I was appointed Chief Deputy, and remained in that capacity through the time Cyril was there.*

At the outset of Steve Zappala's tenure as DA, I was supposed to be something of a mentor to him. In fact, his father had instructed young Steve to look to me if he ever needed advice.

JOE DOMINICK: *I can remember Steve coming over to the office and sitting down, looking for advice from Cyril. And Cyril was willing to advise him. He did it many times.*

"Stevie-Boy," as I like to call him, a newly appointed district attorney, tried to get me to back off when it came to prosecutions of police officers for brutality. I was once quoted in the press accusing him, in my own personal style, of "impudence, arrogance, gall of an unmitigated nature, hubris, and unsurpassed chutzpah that absolutely defies explanation." If it was up to Steve Zappala, there would have been no more coroner's inquests, especially when it came to cases involving the police.

JOE DOMINICK: *Cyril looked at things from a lot of different perspectives. When he gave an opinion, it was well thought-out and based on fact. He had a lot of integrity, and he was always looking to be transparent so that people had an understanding about what was going on. With the inquest system, people could come and sit in the courtroom and listen to the testimony of everyone involved. Some inquests made it very clear that certain police officers should be charged, but Zappala did not go forward. I can think of a situation that took place in one of the residences in the Hill District. Three police officers from the Pittsburgh Housing Authority shot a guy in the back, yet Zappala did not want to prosecute.*

Needless to say, Steve Zappala irritated me. I don't believe that the words "integrity" and "transparency" are in his vocabulary. Beyond that, he is an intellectual midget, and

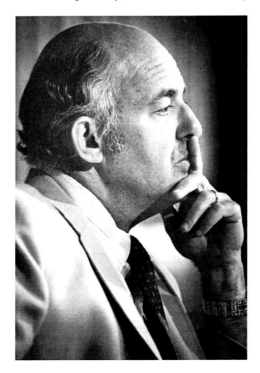

he knows it. In my view, insecurity about not only his intelligence but his legal skills as well, leaves him no choice but to resort to his true nature: that of a narrow-minded, power-hungry bully. For a peek into the dark heart and duplicitous mind of Steve Zappala, Jr., one needs to look no further than the case of Robert Wideman, whose life of crime as a youth led to a decades-long ordeal.

In 1975, Robbie Wideman and two associates lured a man named Nicholas Morena to a meeting in a used-car lot on the South Side of Pittsburgh, promising him a truckload of stolen televisions. Robbie and his partners knew that, by reputation, the owners would buy "hot" goods that they would fence and then sell for profit.

JOHN EDGAR WIDEMAN: *Robbie and his buddies were crooks stealing from crooks. They went to that used-car lot with a van full*

Taking stock, 1985 (*Pittsburgh-Post-Gazette*).

of nothing. They pulled at least one gun on Morena and said, "Give us the money," but Morena wanted to inspect the televisions first. At that point, they had to admit that they had none, and Morena, who they were essentially holding up, either didn't take them seriously or decided that he was going to get the hell out of there, so he ran.

One of Robbie Wideman's partners fired a shot, perhaps accidentally or just trying to scare Morena, depending on whose account you believe. Morena was struck in the shoulder and went down. But he got up and kept running. Robbie and his partners fled the scene and hit the road.

As he traveled west trying to evade capture, Robbie Wideman learned that Morena had died. A few days later, Robbie was apprehended in Colorado, and was then returned to and tried in Pittsburgh. For his role as an accomplice in the robbery of Nicholas Morena, Robbie and one of his associates were convicted of second-degree murder and received life without parole, a mandatory sentence in Pennsylvania for the commission of a felony that results in the death of another person. (Robbie's other associate was convicted of third-degree murder and sentenced to 10 to 20 years in prison.)

Now, here's where the plot thickens. It turned out that Nicholas Morena did not actually die from the gunshot wound he received that night in the used-car lot.

MARK SCHWARTZ: *Morena had been shot, but when he was picked up by an ambulance on a street corner in Pittsburgh, he seemed to be joking around. The ambulance took him to South Side Hospital, which turned him away because they said they didn't have a thoracic surgeon. The ambulance drivers were told to take Morena to Mercy Hospital. So, they did, and when they arrived there, the bandage from Morena's shoulder was removed, blood poured out and he died. But for a chest tube, which was commonly available, Morena would likely have survived.*

Morena's family sued Southside Hospital and two doctors for mishandling the situation by not offering the necessary equipment to the ambulance team to make sure that Morena stayed alive until he reached Mercy Hospital. The suit was successful and the family was paid a large sum of money. But it turned out that the DA at Robbie Wideman's trial did not enter this fact into evidence, nor did he tell Robbie's attorneys.

Nonetheless, Robbie did his time, maturing from the angry, rebellious 24-year-old he was in 1975 into a respectable young man. He kicked heroin, a drug that, in part, fueled his life of crime, and helped other inmates to attain sobriety. He earned an associate's degree in engineering, took courses in computer science, and assisted other inmates with their math studies. When Robbie's lawyers found out about the Morena family's legal settlement, they believed it was cause for a mistrial, or maybe a new trial. Upon reviewing the facts, I told them that I agreed.

JOHN EDGAR WIDEMAN: *My brother's hearing took place in open court and Cyril Wecht was a witness. It was very courageous for him to testify because the atmosphere in Pittsburgh was quite ugly. There was an election coming up and the DA, Steve Zappala, was one of those "Put him in jail and throw away the key" types. He didn't want to hear about releasing a "murderer."*

At the hearing, in 1998, I stepped up and said, in essence, "If I had known, back in the day, what I know now about the shooting, there never would have been a second-degree murder charge. I would not have signed on to that because the victim did not die from the gunshot wound." Nicholas Morena died from medical maltreatment—it's on the record—and the Morena family profited from his death. Even though the case was settled out of court, there were enough records to make this clear. I believed that Robbie Wideman was owed the right to be released pending a decision about a possible second trial.

So, Mark Schwartz, John Wideman and I worked on Robbie's behalf, writing letters, issuing reports and so forth, and it seemed as if he was finally going to be released. On the day that was to occur, the Wideman family had gathered at Robbie's sister's house in Homewood. People were very excited, cooking food and preparing for his homecoming after more than 30 years of incarceration. But not so fast.

JOHN EDGAR WIDEMAN: *The judge had used Cyril's evidence, along with other evidence, to grant Robbie the possibility of a new trial. And my brother was supposedly on his way home when we got a call. Robbie was not coming. He was not going to be released. Steve Zappala had appealed the ruling. We were devastated, particularly because I had stood in the DA's office [with Robbie's lawyer, Mark Schwartz], when Zappala said that he was not going to appeal.*

Minutes before the court shut its door for the day, Stevie-Boy (or perhaps one of his assistants on his behalf) in his infinite malevolence, went to the chambers of Judge James R. McGregor, appealed the Judge's order for a new trial, and had it overturned.

MARK SCHWARTZ: *McGregor, to his death, was very upset about the whole thing. I wanted to hold Zappala in contempt, but all the Judge wanted was an apology, and he couldn't even get that.*

JOHN EDGAR WIDEMAN: *Zappala double-crossed us. My brother never came home that day. And there was a certain amount of animosity directed toward Cyril because he was taking the side of a criminal. He was getting in Zappala's face and interfering in the politics of the District Attorney's upcoming election. Nobody was forgiven; not my brother, and not Cyril Wecht.*

MARK SCHWARTZ: *Cyril was a huge help in the case. We also had Judge Jeffrey A. Manning. As a young DA, Manning prosecuted Robbie Wideman, but had second thoughts about his sentence.*

In fact, Manning wrote a law review article calling the sentencing guidelines for Robbie's crime "draconian" in their call for mandatory life imprisonment without parole for those convicted of murder during the commission of a felony, even if they were not *directly* responsible for the death of another person. Manning joined Mark Schwartz at the Pardon Board hearing and advocated for Robbie Wideman's release.

Twenty years later, in August 2018, for the seventh time, the Pardon Board turned down Robbie's request for release by a vote of 4–1. Frustrated by this, Mark Schwartz went through all the documents again and came up with a Petition to Reconsider. In 2019, the Board voted 5–0 to hear the petition, and then 5–0 to grant Robbie clemency. Pennsylvania Governor Tom Wolf then followed through.

MARK SCHWARTZ: *I decided to use Manning as a witness for the Pardon Board, and it worked.*

Thankfully, today, Robbie Wideman is a free man.

MARK SCHWARTZ: *Steve Zappala cost Robbie Wideman 21 years of freedom. And it wasn't just a matter of having a different view on the matter. He ignored a court order. The Sheriff of Allegheny County said, "Mr. Schwartz, I sent my deputies to get Mr. Wideman, but the jail wouldn't release him because of a call from the DA." He'd never seen anything like that in his career. The question is, did "Baby Zappala" talk to "Daddy Zappala," who was Chief Justice of the Pennsylvania Supreme Court at the time?*

Steve Zappala was consistently in favor of Nicholas Morena, who was a fence for stolen goods. Was there some connection between the Zappalas and the Morenas? Likely, we will never know.

◆ ◆ ◆

KERRY LEWIS: *I knew Cyril because my father ran as a judge and Cyril was in Democratic politics in Allegheny County at the time. He was and remains a highly regarded and intelligent guy. And he's a friendly guy, too, with a lot of charisma. I consulted with him on some medical malpractice cases as an expert. Then I got the Charles Dixon case.*

In December 2002, an incident occurred at a birthday party at Mt. Oliver Fire Hall, where a local black man had perhaps a little too much to drink. He was doing nothing violent or destructive; he was just being disruptive.

Partygoers reported that the man had been causing some trouble at the party by sticking his hand into a bowl of spaghetti at the buffet table. A security guard who was patrolling the party started barking at the man, and the man barked back. In short order, the guard called police from Mt. Oliver and the City of Pittsburgh, because the city literally surrounds Mt. Oliver. A total of 13 officers arrived and the situation quickly escalated.

When police officers attempted to arrest the man, the man's brother, Charles A. Dixon of Altoona, Pennsylvania—a 330-pound, 43-year-old, African American man—intervened, saying something to this effect: "Take it easy on him. He's all right. He's just been drinking a little too much." Before long, Charles Dixon was thrown to the ground, face-first. He was then held down by police and he suffocated because of the pressure.

In this case, I believed strongly that the police officers involved should have been investigated, at the very least. Kerry Lewis told me that one of them had said, "He's turning purple," and another, "Let the nigger die." Some witnesses said that the police officers were using racial slurs while Charles Dixon was on the ground suffering from asphyxiation.

KERRY LEWIS: *There was no brawl. It was merely Charles Dixon being "aggressive" by raising his voice. Charles was a big man but they didn't have to do what they did. There should have been a criminal civil rights case brought by the Attorney General. Somebody should have moved in. But Zappala didn't want it, didn't take any action, and I don't think he referred it. At the time, I asked him and I know that people in the community asked him, but he wasn't interested.*

Over the last thirty or forty years, when it comes to the number of racial incidents between black people and the Pittsburgh-area police, very few officers have been charged, let alone tried.

KERRY LEWIS: *If you're a cop in Pittsburgh or Allegheny County, you are operating in an environment that allows you to be careless in your conduct, to push situations to the edge, as far as the prosecution is concerned. It may even result in criminal activity by law enforcement, justified in the name of maintaining "law and order," especially when it comes to black people.*

TONY NORMAN: *In the Dixon case, Zappala really did represent very "establishment" thinking about a crime against a black person. I've always seen Cyril's willingness to stand up for black defendants as honorable. He has often provided the rationale that black families need to move forward with their own opposition to the official narrative. The Dixon case is a case in point.*

RONALD FREEMAN: *There were times when Cyril said things and made decisions that the police didn't like but, having been involved in the system and understanding how things worked, I thought he was down-the-middle, pretty much. I have no problem with what he did. We discussed it all the time, in person and on the phone. He did an excellent job as Coroner.*

Plaudits notwithstanding, my advice to black people in Pittsburgh: Don't get involved with the police. Keep your hands up and your mouths shut. Trust me, you can't win, especially with a man like Steve Zappala as the DA. Zappala sees himself as a "tough guy." He is mean-spirited and, in my opinion, is a tremendously insecure person with a borderline sociopathic personality.

Once, in conversation, I asked then–Allegheny County Executive Dan Onorato if he had ever been "muscled" by Zappala. Dan told me that the two were not friends, and that Zappala was none too happy with him. In fact, he had "suggested" that Onorato turn the reins of the Allegheny County Police over to the District Attorney's Office. If that would have happened, the force would have ceased to be the independent entity it had always been, under the control of the county. Onorato refused to accede to the DA's wishes. But, as further evidence of what I perceived to be his increasing megalomania, Steve Zappala made a play to take over the Coroner's Office, too.

JOE DOMINICK: *Cyril did his job effectively and was probably the best medical examiner the county ever had, or will have. The situation came about because Steve Zappala didn't like what Cyril was doing [especially when it came to inquests involving police officers], and he wanted control of the County Crime Lab.*

TIM UHRICH: *I remember one time that Steve wanted to have a meeting with us. He brought one or two of his people over to the Coroner's Office and proceeded to give us his "control" speech, about how he couldn't be an effective DA if he didn't have total control over the county's entire criminal justice system. Cyril listened to him patiently and responded, "I hear what you're saying, Steve, but what's really important to me is the independence of this office."*

Tim Uhrich recalls Zappala's follow-up to my response as something akin to the following: "Listen here, old man; you're on your way out. I'm in charge now and must have control of everything." Again, I said "No." And you don't just say "no" to Steve Zappala. It was a sign of things to come.

Ultimately, Zappala is a political coward. He is lazy, both intellectually and physically. That's why he has remained DA rather than moving on to a higher governmental office. In 2005, the Democratic Party was virtually willing to hand him the nomination to run for Pennsylvania Attorney General—the office was open—but Zappala declined.

WILLIAM ROBINSON: *If Zappala ever plans to run for another office, he's going to have to be held accountable. I don't know anything about his lawyering skills, though I haven't heard any positive stories about them. And I don't know what case he could make other than, "I've helped to maintain the status quo, race-wise, in Allegheny County. I've done things with which the black community has disagreed. And I've done a lot of things with which the police have agreed. So, I'm your guy." He would be hard-pressed to run for a statewide office successfully.*

In 2016, when Zappala finally did decide to run for Attorney General, he got clobbered, and I was happy to help that happen. I encouraged Josh Shapiro, an attorney and politician from Eastern Pennsylvania, to run and then strongly supported him in both the primary and general elections. Zappala apparently thought it would be a "cake walk," so he mounted a lackluster and unconvincing campaign, and Shapiro beat him soundly in the Democratic primary.

JOSH SHAPIRO: *Cyril Wecht was the first public person that I asked for support, and I was honored that he backed me. He gave me a perspective on my opponent that virtually no one else could have, and his reach is tremendous. Cyril was able to give me a foothold in Western Pennsylvania that I could build from. He gave me credibility early on in the process with voters. And he was relentless in his campaigning on my behalf. I know that my victory is due, in part, to Cyril's advocacy. There were a handful of endorsements that really mattered in my race, and Cyril Wecht's was one of them.*

Today, Zappala is comfortable where he is. He won't ever run for another office and is not going anywhere, that is unless his all-powerful family can finagle a judicial appointment for him.

◆ ◆ ◆

With the notion of total control seemingly off the table, another internal issue began to fester between the DA and the Coroner's Office, and it metastasized into nothing less than a political showdown between Steve Zappala and me over my ongoing insistence that open inquests be conducted for all death cases involving police officers. In conducting these open inquests, I had fueled a turf war with the DA. Before long, he had gone from being merely annoying to potentially dangerous. As Coroner, I had traditional inquisitorial power, and I used it to the fullest extent, which I believed was the right thing to do. But Zappala was very unhappy about the situation and became increasingly hostile towards me. Over time, a split occurred between Zappala and me, and it kept widening.

Like the majority of his predecessors in the Allegheny County District Attorney's Office, Steve Zappala would do whatever he had to do to protect the police. Since his appointment in 1997, he has cultivated their support and has always been tight with them. In his fantasies, he is now the bad-ass cop he never was, so he had to manage police-related incidents very, very carefully.

In two decades as the DA of Pennsylvania's second-biggest county, Steve Zappala hasn't prosecuted more than a handful of police officers. After all, for him—and, to be fair, for most district attorneys, no matter what jurisdiction—the police are akin to his arms and legs. He works with them and thinks of them in terms of the political support they offer. Given Pittsburgh's under-publicized but serious racial problems, Zappala's love affair with the city's police proved to be a flashpoint between Allegheny County and the local black community, and between Steve Zappala and me. Soon, our wrangling over cases involving the police would turn very ugly.

What brought the situation to a crisis was the aforementioned Charles Dixon case. And little did I know that my life would be turned upside-down by the S.O.B. in the DA's Office. In my opinion, the arrest of Mr. Dixon was unwarranted. Remember, we are talking about his brother sticking his hand into a bowl of spaghetti. That was the "crime." If 13 cops couldn't handle such a situation without piling on and suffocating a man, there is something seriously wrong with their training.

In discussing the case, I drew comparisons between the cause of Dixon's death and that of Jonny Gammage, an African American man who, in 1995, was visiting Pittsburgh from Syracuse, New York, and was beaten to death by police for "driving erratically" in a predominantly white suburb. I was not Allegheny County Coroner at the time of the incident but, after I was re-elected and returned to the post in 1996, I had the opportunity to testify at the ensuing trials, of which there were three. (I caused a mistrial in the initial go-around by suggesting that one of the defendants take the stand and explain *exactly* what had happened to the young businessman.) I contended that the local police, once again, had over-reacted and used excessive force on Charles Dixon.

JOE DOMINICK: *When Cyril made a statement about a particular case, he was rarely wrong. I can't recall any instance in which he made a decision that turned out to be anything but the right one, even though he sometimes was met with a lot of opposition. Cyril was emotional with some of his statements, but he was on target.*

Zappala and I talked and talked about the Dixon case. We even took the time to officially re-enact the incident. But the relationship between us became increasingly acrimonious until it reached a point at which we ceased to talk with one another at all. In time, the issue of whether or not the Coroner's Office had the right to conduct open inquests in death cases involving police officers went before Judge Jeffrey A. Manning, and Zappala didn't even attend the court proceedings. Instead, he sent an assistant to speak for him. He considered me his enemy at that point. So, he went to work, fishing around for something—anything—with which to hang me.

Charles Dixon's death was clearly a homicide due to positional asphyxiation, and

I recommended that charges be filed against the police officers involved. But after reviewing my findings, Steve Zappala decided to go even a step less than did former DA Bob Colville in his half-hearted (and ultimately unsuccessful) prosecution of the officers in the Jonny Gammage case: He decided to press *no charges at all* against the police officers who caused Charles Dixon's death. Not only was I offended by Zappala's lack of respect for my findings, I was outraged by his failure of duty.

As time wore on, it became clear that Steve Zappala had no intention of changing his course as related to the case of Charles Dixon. So, frustrated and realizing that they would never have their day in criminal court, Dixon's relatives decided to pursue a civil action against Allegheny County for "wrongful death."

According to the *Pittsburgh Post-Gazette*, the family's suit claimed that the officers used a "swarming" technique to arrest Dixon, in which they grabbed his arms and legs, threw him to the ground and held him there while they applied pressure to his torso. After Dixon lapsed into unconsciousness, they left him for 10 minutes without performing cardiopulmonary resuscitation. Paramedics performed CPR when they arrived and took Dixon to Mercy Hospital, where he died 48 hours later without regaining consciousness. The suit also suggested that the actions of the officers, all of whom were white, were motivated by race.

> KERRY LEWIS: *I filed a civil rights case [on behalf of the Dixon family] and wrote to Cyril at his private office asking him to prepare a report describing and explaining positional asphyxiation. Cyril was never hired to be a witness in the case. The Coroner's Office had done the pathology report, so Cyril couldn't be a witness because one of the pathologists in his office did the job.*

As the Dixon family prepared for their civil trial against Allegheny County, in my capacity as an employee of Wecht Pathology Associates, my private consulting firm, I agreed to provide the report that Kerry Lewis requested. In reaction to that report, Steve Zappala went ballistic.

> KERRY LEWIS: *One day, I got a phone call from Zappala, who wanted to know about Cyril's report. "Did Cyril write this report from the Coroner's Office?" he asked. I said, "No. My letter of request was addressed to Cyril at his private office, and he wrote back on his private stationery." A few months later, I was subpoenaed to produce that report, and I did. When I brought it to the [assistant] district attorney who was handling the case at the time, I went into the courtroom and reiterated: "This report was done by Dr. Wecht's private practice, and I'm going to object to testify on it. He was an expert hired by the plaintiff." On the basis of that report came Cyril's whole federal case.*

Lazy person that he is, Zappala couldn't understand, given that I was already 72 years old, how I could possibly have had time to prepare the report for the Dixon family, while shouldering a huge workload as Allegheny County Coroner. Well, unlike most civil servants, 70–90-hour weeks were not unusual for me. I'm an ambitious and hard-working kid from the Lower Hill. My county job didn't pay all that much and I had a mortgage to meet. Every evening, with the exception of most Sundays, I would head home for dinner and a little family time. Then afterward, off I would go to work on my ever-increasing private caseload. It was a fast-paced and rigorous schedule, but it paid the bills, and it was interesting.

JERRY MCDEVITT: *What Cyril said about the Dixon case was correct, and here's what Zappala did to him for that. The opinion that Cyril prepared for the Dixon family's civil attorney, stating the cause and manner of Charles Dixon's death and all the rest, had to be typed, of course, and it was—on a county computer—by Cyril's secretary, Eileen Young. To Zappala, that constituted "use of county resources for private purposes." Believe it or not, the inconsequential fact that the Dixon opinion was typed on a county computer is what started Cyril's whole legal fiasco.*

Federal Trial Part I

Choose a Victim, Invent a Crime

If one considers the political landscape of the first decade of the 21st century, the United States was a risky place for liberal Democrats like me. In 2001, the September 11 terror attacks had reduced the World Trade Center to rubble in lower Manhattan. Fear of similar events happening on American soil spread, and many U.S. citizens decided that they were willing to cede more authority to the federal government to keep themselves safe. Collective fear was the best thing that ever happened for the administration of George W. Bush. It was its stock in trade. But as Benjamin Franklin once said, "Those who would give up essential liberty to purchase a little temporary safety, deserve neither liberty nor safety." And that's just what we got—neither.

At the time, the nation was mired in wars in both Afghanistan and Iraq, conflicts in which young American men and women were dying nearly every day, along with loads of Afghani and Iraqi citizens. But in the corridors of power in the nation's capital, and in cities large and small throughout the nation, the Republican Party had its sights set on more than "radical Islam." Indeed, it was a rather poorly kept secret that one plank of the GOP's unofficial national campaign strategy was to smear prominent Democrats by way of political prosecution. If Republican candidates couldn't prevail at the ballot box, at least they could keep their opponents' hands (and purse strings) tied with bad publicity and the risk of legal jeopardy.

In the minds of those who believed in the *modus operandi* of the Bush administration, it was the duty of all conservative-leaning, Republican-appointed U.S. Attorneys to further the GOP's cause. As the years between 2001 and 2005 slipped by with no successful acts of terror reported in the "Homeland," preventing terrorism was no longer the nation's top law enforcement priority. It was replaced by a focus on public corruption, and the U.S. Department of Justice seized upon it.

To fill the wing-tips of the departing right-wing ideologue John Ashcroft (he of the ignominious "Patriot Act"), in February 2005, President Bush appointed a new Attorney General: a younger, more aggressive, and not-too-bright fellow–Texan named Alberto Gonzales. Not surprisingly, Gonzales arrived in Washington with an agenda. He chose to begin his tenure with an assessment of his troops, some of whom he found wanting. Before long, Gonzales sought the resignation of a host of U.S.

Attorneys who (as the public would later learn) weren't prosecuting individuals that the conservative Republican administration thought should be prosecuted; namely, Democrats.

At just 42 years of age, Mary Beth Buchanan, the U.S. Attorney for the Western District of Pennsylvania, was the first woman and youngest person ever to hold a U.S. Attorney's position in Pennsylvania's history. She had served as Director of the Executive Office for U.S. Attorneys when "Bush's brain," Karl Rove, and then–Attorney General Ashcroft hatched the plan to fire Republican U.S. Attorneys for failing to prosecute Democrats with sufficient partisan zeal.

Back in Pittsburgh, District Attorney Stephen Zappala, still fuming over what he saw as my interference in the case of Charles Dixon, decided to gain leverage by launching an investigation into whether or not I was using county resources to carry out my private work. How could a man like me, in his 70s, accomplish so much in his private practice, unless he was cutting corners on the county side?

Some time passed but, having been harassed and hounded once by the authorities in a legal hassle at the local level, for the first time in 25 years I began to perceive the rumblings of some potential trouble again. I had heard some things that concerned me, so I asked my lawyer at the time, David Armstrong, to call around and see if I was being investigated for any reason.

David called First Assistant U.S. Attorney Robert Cessar to ask if his office was investigating me. I was in the room with David when he placed the call. Cessar said he knew of no such investigation, but said that he would check into it. When he called back, he said simply that there was an investigation, but it wasn't being conducted by his office. "It's the FBI," Cessar told us. We were shocked. Both David Armstrong and I believed that Cessar's response indicated that the U.S. Attorney's Office knew nothing about an investigation targeting me—initially. But with the sights of the FBI locked upon me, I knew that it wouldn't be long until the young, hyper-partisan U.S. Attorney for the Western District of Pennsylvania smelled blood, too.

In April 2005, the FBI conducted publicly unannounced but media-leaked raids on both the Allegheny County Coroner's Office and my private office at Wecht Pathology Associates, seizing public and private documents, ostensibly related to my conduct of business on both fronts. And, on January 20, 2006, U.S. Attorney Mary Beth Buchanan filed an 84-count felony indictment against me for theft, fraud and other abuses of office. She did it in grand style at a news conference in Pittsburgh, during which she took pleasure in enumerating the counts leveled against me.

Not long after the announcement, my attorneys, Dick Thornburgh and Mark Rush from the law firm of K&L Gates (two devout and active Republicans, incidentally) arranged a meeting at the U.S. Attorney's Office in Pittsburgh to try, as defense lawyers do, to talk sense to the prosecution. As a former U.S. Attorney and former Attorney General of the United States, Dick Thornburgh knew what a criminal case looked like, and mine was not a criminal case. With his customary decorum, Dick proceeded to outline for the unquestionably green and undoubtedly ambitious U.S. Attorney what he believed were the shortcomings of the government's case against me.

RICHARD THORNBURGH: *Most of the charging counts alleged nickel-and-dime transgressions which were converted into federal felony charges.*

Some of those allegations involved, for example: the use of county fax machines for personal business, such as the transmission of my *curriculum vitae* and fee schedule to a local public defender seeking my assistance, and an executed contract for a teaching engagement. Other allegations included unreimbursed postage charges for mailing histological slides to attorneys who had consulted me in Black Lung cases, and expense billing errors in invoices mailed to my private clients. A number of felony counts derived from alleged improper billing for use of a county car while traveling to outlying counties to assist local prosecutors and coroners.

RICHARD THORNBURGH: *Astonishingly, the government's own evidence indicated that an audit of the billings of Dr. Wecht to the counties in question showed them to be 99.99 percent accurate, a record that was nonetheless turned into 37 felony counts covering a very small sum of money.*

But U.S. Attorney Buchanan and her brash and ambitious assistant Stephen S. Stallings, who also was present at the meeting with Thornburgh and Rush, along with representatives from the FBI, would have none of it. They insisted that the government had a bona fide corruption case against me. I was a notable Democrat, so there was no way to dissuade them.

MARK RUSH: *It was clear from the start that they were committed to prosecuting Cyril.*

Even so, Thornburgh and Rush walked Buchanan, Stallings, *et al.*, through each and every reason why the government's case was flawed and would not lead to a conviction. Buchanan did some cursory countering but, primarily, she and her colleagues just sat and listened.

MARK RUSH: *They didn't want to tip their hand, so they didn't say much.*

At the meeting's conclusion, Thornburgh summed things up. Looking directly at Mary Beth Buchanan, he said, "Everyone in this room will regret it greatly if you prosecute Cyril Wecht," after which Stephen Stallings retorted, rather disrespectfully, "Are you threatening us?"

Enter K&L Gates trial attorney Jerry McDevitt, who assumed the role of lead counsel for my case.

JERRY MCDEVITT: *If Cyril had come to me and said he wanted to plead to something, I would have told him that he had the wrong guy. I'm not a plea lawyer. But Cyril never wanted to talk about a plea bargain, and we never did.*

So strong is McDevitt in his antipathy toward plea bargaining that he has never read in full the federal sentencing guidelines because, in his estimation, "All they do is make lawyers afraid to try cases because of fear of what might happen if they do." Jerry had represented clients in federal trials on three occasions, and not one of them had been convicted on even a single count.

MARK RUSH: *Cyril was confronted by all the power, authority, and weight of the federal government. He had to win on all counts. If the jury decided that the government hadn't proven its case on all 84 counts, but maybe it did on a couple of them, and found Cyril guilty on those while acquitting him on the others, it still would have had a devastating impact on his life.*

In fact, I would have lost, almost certainly, my right to practice law and, who knows, maybe even my medical license, too. So, it seemed that Mary Beth Buchanan had succeeded, at least partially, in her mission to cast a well-known local Democrat in a negative light during an election year.

JERRY MCDEVITT: *The number of charges in these types of cases is meaningless to me. The government's game is to throw as much as it can at a defendant in hope that a jury will convict on at least one or two charges. For a prosecutor, that spells victory. But as a defense attorney, even if my client is cleared of all but one charge, it is a defeat for me. So, these cases are much tougher battles for us than they are for federal prosecutors. And they become personal.*

According to Mark Rush (who would, ultimately, assist Jerry McDevitt with my defense), at Buchanan's notorious news conference announcing the charges against me, the U.S. Attorney literally waved around her indictment for its "shock and awe effect." But, he continued, when it came time to prepare for trial…

MARK RUSH: *They quickly realized that their indictment was just as we described it to them: flawed, and fatally so.*

From a legal standpoint, it was clear to Rush that the U.S. Attorney's Office had composed the indictment to be little more than a damning press release and did not think about how it was going to try the case. In Rush's view, to say that the government over-charged is an understatement of gross proportions. The case against me was one in which a specific individual was targeted for investigation and prosecution.

MARK RUSH: *It wasn't as if there was a course of conduct that was clearly illegal and, therefore, worthy of indictment. Cyril himself was targeted, and the government attempted to create facts that could be woven together to warrant an indictment.*

Dick Thornburgh echoed Rush's assessment. Mine was not the type of case normally constituting a federal corruption action against a local official.

RICHARD THORNBURGH: *None of the traditional indicia of public corruption were present. There was no allegation that Cyril solicited or received a bribe or kickback. And there was no allegation that he traded on a conflict of interest in conducting the affairs of his elected office.*

Instead, the prosecution sought to use unprecedented theories to convert into federal felonies a mixed bag of alleged violations of home rule charters, county codes, and even state ethics rules. In the process, Mary Beth Buchanan and her staff were stretching the bounds of federal law beyond the breaking point.

RICHARD THORNBURGH: *Many of the alleged underlying violations didn't even carry state mandated penalties, yet they were utilized as a vehicle for a federal felony prosecution which branded Cyril as a corrupt public servant. The U.S. Attorney also proclaimed, among other things, that Cyril had, in her words, "literally" provided un- claimed cadavers to a local Catholic university in exchange for free lab space.*

The charge alleged that, while teaching at Carlow University in Pittsburgh, I traded unclaimed bodies from the County Morgue to the school in exchange for space to con- duct private autopsies. With that, I was labeled a "body snatcher" in the press, and a media feeding-frenzy ensued.

The press ate up the body-snatching nonsense. Mark Rush confided to me that he was incredulous at the contention that Carlow University, with a nun, Sister Grace Ann Geibel, at the helm, had engaged in a conspiracy to trade human corpses for the use of its laboratory.

MARK RUSH: *It was so crazy. I asked that they tell us what witnesses they were going to call to say that this had happened, but they never did. It was just another unsubstantiated smear against Cyril, and a pretty effective one, with the press, anyway.*

JERRY MCDEVITT: *The initial publicity surrounding Cyril's indictment was unbelievably cold-hearted and nasty. The newspapers published cartoons of him pushing corpses and trading money. It was as ugly as ugly can get.*

Through pretrial motions, I had been represented well by Dick Thornburgh in hope that the prominent and well-respected Republican could convince another Re- publican, U.S. Attorney Mary Beth Buchanan, to drop the case against me. Dick's ef- forts, unfortunately, came to naught. But as the investigation into my practices, both public and private, proceeded, on October 23, 2007, Dick Thornburgh, a proud and staunch Republican if there ever was one, was called to testify by the U.S. House of Representatives at a hearing before the Committee on the Judiciary about "Allegations of Selective Prosecution: The Erosion of Public Confidence in Our Federal Justice Sys- tem." The House panel was investigating the then-burgeoning U.S. Attorneys firing scandal.

Dick had spent nearly half of his career in the U.S. Department of Justice: begin- ning in 1969 as the U.S. Attorney for the Western District of Pennsylvania, where he earned a reputation for being tough on organized crime; and from 1988 to 1991 as U.S. Attorney General under President George H.W. Bush. (He also served as Governor of Pennsylvania for two terms, from 1979 to 1987.) Thornburgh testified that he was convinced that I had been targeted politically. His testimony was replete with warnings about how such misguided actions only served to erode public confidence in our fed- eral judicial system.

"*In addition to Dr. Wecht's high profile in the area of forensic pathology,*" said Thorn- burgh before the U.S. House Committee, "*he has always been a contentious, outspo- ken, highly critical and highly visible Democratic figure in Western Pennsylvania. He was the perfect target for a Republican U.S. Attorney who was trying to curry favor with the Department of Justice, which had demonstrated that, if you play by its rules, you will advance.*"

Without a doubt, I believe that Mary Beth Buchanan manufactured a case against me, a prominent member of the Democratic Party, as a vehicle for her professional advancement.

Jerry McDevitt: *Mary Beth told everybody who would listen that she hoped to ride the Wecht prosecution into a federal judgeship. And by doing so, she figured that she would be able to make some "brownie-points" with the Bush White House and Department of Justice. Whatever it took, she was going to do their bidding.*

Albeit high profile, the case against me was not the only contemporaneous and politically suspicious investigation and prosecution in Western Pennsylvania. For example, Buchanan also conducted highly visible grand jury investigations of Tom Murphy, who was pressured to resign as Mayor of Pittsburgh, and Pete DeFazio, who was forced out of his position as Sheriff of Allegheny County. Buchanan also prosecuted several other employees of the Sheriff's Office.

Richard Thornburgh: *It should be noted that, of the U.S. Attorney's two previous major public prosecutions of Democrats, one resulted in a misdemeanor plea, and the other resulted in no plea with an alternative resolution.*

But these investigations were splashed all over newspapers and TV running up to the 2006 elections. All were "page-one" material. And the "scandals," whether true or simply implied, were poison to Democratic political candidates. Much damage was done. But compared to the Murphy and DeFazio investigations, my prosecution would be the "big one." The stakes were high. To save face and move up the ladder at Justice, Mary Beth Buchanan desperately needed to convict a Democrat, at any cost.

Buchanan was, by all accounts, a person of modest educational background whose legal acumen and level of experience could be described most generously as "limited." In fact, up until my case, her only claim to fame was having snagged a member of the blue blood Buchanan family of Pittsburgh—as in the gargantuan and prestigious law firm Buchanan Ingersoll—as her husband.

Tim Uhrich: *Mary Beth was a non-factor for her entire life. She was a second-level prosecutor who, due to connections I'm sure, was able to jump over everybody to the U.S. Attorney's Office. And she was so out of her depth in that role that it was embarrassing, even to her colleagues, and I knew a bunch of them. But she was a darling of the right-wing conservatives because she would do things that no other self-respecting U.S. Attorney would do.*

After fifty years as a doctor, lawyer and politician, I had come to know a bit about how people think. When a huge number of charges—84 in my case—are leveled against any prominent official and are trumpeted in bold newspaper headlines and on TV, many people figure that at least some of them must be true.

From the outset, my lead defense attorney, Jerry McDevitt, was concerned about the scope of the indictment. Eighty-four counts are a lot to handle, for any legal team. Then, curiously, in January 2008, just two weeks prior to the start of court proceedings in my case, and after I had already spent a mountain of cash over a three-year period preparing to answer all charges, the prosecution elected to withdraw 43 of the 84 counts it had leveled, charges that were then dismissed with prejudice.

JERRY MCDEVITT: *It was very unusual. The judge in the case had to approve all of this and, of course, he was all for it because it simplified the trial for him.*

To understand just what happened to me ultimately in the years between 2005 and 2008, one has to start at the beginning. I believe that the legal inferno that would come to engulf much of my life and consume much of my money began with a small brush fire, intentionally set, in my beloved hometown.

To this day, I believe that the Allegheny County District Attorney's Office produced the spark for the federal investigation of my business affairs in a vindictive attempt to set my life and career ablaze for not only challenging the authority of Steve Zappala, who wanted me out of the way as he pushed to consolidate his power, but also as payback for my unwillingness to dispense with potential cases against Pittsburgh area police officers accused of brutality.

Interestingly, before I was indicted, a message was communicated to my lawyer, David Armstrong. In essence, Armstrong was told, "If Cyril agrees not to apply for the Medical Examiner's position, all of this will go away." I was told that this message was sent from Steve Zappala. I believe that, after receiving no response from me, Zappala or his agents contacted the FBI and stoked the flames of a federal investigation into my so-called "public-private conflict of interest" by way of a nefarious bully named Bradley Orsini, a career FBI agent who had been, in essence, exiled to the Bureau's Pittsburgh office from Newark. Orsini was the perfect man to carry out the plan that Zappala had hatched. He took the initiative to push it at the federal level, thus giving Mary Beth Buchanan a golden opportunity to prosecute a notable local Democrat.

It remains unclear whether or not Zappala and Orsini knew each other before my case. It is also unclear who initiated their interaction. Did Zappala contact the FBI? Or did Orsini come to Pittsburgh and go to the DA?

MARK RUSH: *Did this begin with Steve Zappala? Cyril believes that it did. What we do know is that meetings were held between Zappala and the FBI about the Wecht case, so I think the genesis came from the county, and it may very well have been over the relationship between the Coroner's inquest powers and the powers of the DA. I know Zappala wanted to dramatically limit or even eliminate the Coroner's power to hold open inquests.*

Prosecutors in the U.S. Attorney's Office, who had an ongoing relationship with the DA in Pittsburgh (largely because of trading off drug-related cases), saw their opportunity. And again, I believe that they picked up the case against me for both political reasons and professional ambition.

At times, all of this trouble with Mary Beth Buchanan seemed strange because, up to that point, my relationship with her had been cordial. She had accepted a position on the advisory board of the Cyril H. Wecht Institute of Forensic Science and Law, which I had established at Duquesne University in Pittsburgh in the fall of 2000. She had even invited me to take the stage with her and then–U.S. Attorney General John Ashcroft when Allegheny County received a large federal grant to upgrade its law enforcement system, part of which was to go to the Coroner's Office. So why would Mary Beth Buchanan so readily join in Steve Zappala's bid to nail me?

JERRY McDEVITT: *Mary Beth had a situation in which one prominent Democrat was handing her another to prosecute, which is exactly what Zappala did. A partisan Republican like her would run with that in a "New York minute."*

By the time K&L Gates got involved in my case, I had already been indicted and was the ongoing subject of sensational and lurid press coverage with headlines that screamed of "rampant fraud," and "body-snatching." Jerry McDevitt, a crusty, no-nonsense man of action, decided that he would make a run at Buchanan himself in an effort to try and stop the madness before it went any further. So, soon after taking on the case, McDevitt called Mary Beth Buchanan.

JERRY McDEVITT: *I'd never spoken to her before, but I told her that I would be representing Cyril at trial, and that I'd like to sit down and speak with her about the case which, incidentally, I thought was a "crock of shit."*

To McDevitt's surprise, Buchanan agreed to meet with him at a Starbucks in the William Penn Hotel, in downtown Pittsburgh, after which, coffee in hand, they moved to a local park to talk.

JERRY McDEVITT: *It was interesting because usually U.S. Attorneys want you to come to their offices so that they're in a power position. Anyway, we sat for three hours, and my first impression of Mary Beth was that I liked her. She was flirtatious in a touchy-feely kind of way.*

In any case, Jerry gave the young U.S. Attorney a seasoned trial lawyer's perspective of her case.

JERRY McDEVITT: *"Number one," I said, "I don't know what you know about your FBI agent, but you've got some major problems with him." Orsini was well-known in Newark and they ran him out of town. She pretended not to know anything about it. Then I told her, "Mary Beth, when it comes to this body-snatching thing, you are way out of line. You haven't even spoken with the nun who runs the university. How can you make that kind of charge without talking to Sister Grace Ann at Carlow?"*

As the conversation wore on, it became clear that common ground would not be found, but a strange and perhaps portentous event occurred. A pigeon swooped down over the heads of the two attorneys and dropped its payload on Mary Beth Buchanan's cheek.

JERRY McDEVITT: *I told her, "You know, Mary Beth, that was one of Cyril's pigeons."*

From that point on, every time Jerry McDevitt encountered Mary Beth Buchanan on the street, she'd call out to him, "Cyril has to plead 'guilty' to something," to which he always responded, "Forget it, Mary Beth. He's not going to ruin his career to make yours."

Any prosecution of me, while delectable for a self-promoting true-believer like Mary Beth Buchanan, would have its problems, and the professional history and reputation of lead FBI agent Brad Orsini would be one of them. Just how an utter reprobate such as Orsini was able to elude the screening processes in both the offices of the DA and U.S. Attorney without being found out and dismissed, nobody can answer. But he did. And the situation regarding me, as laid out by Steve Zappala, was just perfect for Orsini's purposes. Frankly speaking, both Jerry McDevitt and Mark Rush were shocked that Brad Orsini was still working for the FBI at all.

> MARK RUSH: *From what we had heard, he was already in his position in Pittsburgh before his personnel file got here. Once it arrived, it was too late. He was already on the job.*

Fortunately, Mark Rush had learned about Orsini's checkered past through his work with an FBI agent on another case in New Jersey.

> MARK RUSH: *I can't recall how it came up. I may have been talking about the Wecht case and mentioned the name "Orsini." When I did, the agent looked at me and asked, "Do you mean Brad Orsini?" I said, "Yes." She said, "We were stationed together in Newark. Do you know about his past?" I didn't—and she was very forthcoming about it.*

In time, my attorneys would learn much about Brad Orsini's numerous disciplinary problems while he was an agent in the FBI's office in Newark, New Jersey. After some wrangling, Mark Rush was able to acquire Orsini's personnel file, and it was clear that he was going to have tremendous credibility issues, if and when he took the stand at my trial.

> MARK RUSH: *The man had so many disciplinary actions taken against him that it became very apparent that he was not going to be able to be the "summary," if you will, case agent who would wrap up things for a jury. Brad Orsini had just too much baggage to be relied upon.*

Reporter Jason Cato, in the *Pittsburgh Tribune-Review*, reported that "Orsini had been investigated by the FBI for seven infractions that led to a demotion and two suspensions without pay." Former colleagues in the Bureau's Newark office described the man as "abrasive and self-centered." One former supervisor characterized him as a "bully."

According to the *Trib*, "…the Office of Professional Responsibility (OPR), the department which investigates wrongdoing by agents, initiated four investigations into Orsini's behavior between 1997 and 2000." Those investigations, which were consolidated into one case, found that (1) Orsini engaged in a prohibited sexual relationship with another agent for nearly two years; (2) threatened a subordinate who he believed told superiors about said relationship; (3) damaged government property by punching holes in office walls with his fists and breaking chairs; and (4) made unprofessional and insensitive "homophobic remarks" while joking around with other agents in the office. "For those transgressions," the *Trib* reported, "Orsini was demoted from a supervisor's role within the Newark public corruption squad to a street agent working narcotics investigations in an outlying field office. He was also suspended without pay for 30 days, placed on probation for one year and forced to undergo sensitivity training. That investigation also found that Orsini violated bureau procedures by signing other agents' initials to interview reports in 1993 and 1994. Orsini told investigators that he did not know how many times he had done so, but said he did it only because 'it was a convenience and a shortcut,' according to the reports. In 1998, Orsini was suspended for five days without pay for falsifying chain of custody forms and evidence labels by, again, signing other agents' names to the documents. Investigators found that Orsini committed these infractions between May 1995 and January 1997. Both times he was reprimanded and Orsini was warned that future infractions could result in his dismissal."

Orsini transferred to the Pittsburgh FBI office in 2005, just in time to make my life miserable. While neither of my lawyers—McDevitt nor Rush—could confirm conclusively Steve Zappala's role in initiating the investigation, we all quickly recognized the dark shadow of Brad Orsini and became concerned that my prosecution involved more opportunism than justice. Playing a major role in convicting me of public corruption would be Orsini's ticket to rehabilitating himself within the ranks of the FBI.

According to the OPR's own investigative conclusion, it was impossible to determine the full extent of the taint on all the evidence Orsini falsified. In short order, however, McDevitt would learn all he would need to know about how the government was planning to play the game of *U.S. v. Wecht* when it came to their "star" witness. The U.S. Attorney's Office filed what McDevitt called "the infamous Document 60," which exposed the whole fighting plan of its case.

As he prepared for trial, reviewing motions that had been filed for my case on the court's electronic filing system, McDevitt stumbled upon a heretofore unknown "motion to seal" submitted by the government. "What is this?" he thought. The next day, he was due to appear for the first time before U.S. District Court Judge Arthur J. Schwab, who was selected to hear my case, to do some prep work and scheduling.

At the end of the session, McDevitt approached Judge Schwab to ask about the mysterious Document 60, of which he had not received a copy. Schwab simply replied that Jerry wouldn't be getting one. "But how am I supposed to respond to a motion that the prosecution has made if I don't get to review it?" he asked, but the Judge brushed off his question. "Surely," McDevitt thought, "Judge Schwab was not going to allow the government to file secret documents with him during a criminal case." Or was he?

The fact that Arthur Schwab was a political and philosophical bedfellow of the ultra-right-wing and, at the time, extremely powerful U.S. Senator from Pennsylvania Rick Santorum, didn't worry McDevitt at first, even though Santorum had gone to the mat by threatening to block every federal appointment to the bench that came before him if Schwab was not approved.

Initially, McDevitt thought that Document 60 might have been a simple request to continue the grand jury or something similar, which might have been legitimate. In truth, what Buchanan had done was, the day after McDevitt told her that she had problems with her FBI witness, she filed a secret motion with Judge Schwab containing nine pages of legal argument as to why a series of FBI reports detailing Brad Orsini's disciplinary problems within the Bureau should not be considered in the Wecht case.

JERRY McDEVITT: *Orsini could have been charged with crimes, and the prosecution was asking the judge for permission not to turn over evidence of his misconduct to us.*

Why a U.S. District Judge would participate in such a bald-faced scheme remains a mystery. It was clearly improper. Schwab should have immediately ordered the prosecution to turn over all FBI reports regarding Brad Orsini to my team. But this was only the beginning of our problems with Arthur J. Schwab.

Fortunately, Jerry McDevitt didn't think Buchanan knew much about trying cases, or about how cases play out at trial. Like Mark Rush, he got the feeling that neither she nor her staff even understood the charges that they had leveled against me or their weaknesses, from a legal standpoint.

Jerry McDevitt continued his due diligence in the case by reviewing the search warrants that had been executed, and he knew that, on their face, they were invalid.

JERRY McDEVITT: *They hadn't been particularized. The authorities have to tell the person who is to be searched what they're searching for, specifically.*

At the time, I was in the process of relocating my private office and, as a result, boxes of private files were being housed temporarily in the Allegheny County Coroner's Office. It was easier for me to work on all my cases, public and private, there.

JERRY McDEVITT: *They tried to make this look like an act of obstruction, because it was Zappala's investigation and, to him, Cyril was trying to get rid of evidence.*

According to Jerry McDevitt, the warrants in my case were so vague that the agents who were charged with search and seizure were left scratching their heads when they confronted my mass of records.

JERRY McDEVITT: *When they showed up at Cyril's private office, there were still hundreds of boxes of documents there, ready to be moved. Which ones were supposed to be searched? Not knowing, they literally started going through every box in the place.*

Ultimately, FBI agent Orsini, who was working the search at the Coroner's Office, was asked by his subordinates, "What are we supposed to take?" He told them, "When you open up a box, if any document has Eileen Young's name on it, take that box." The problem was, the government hadn't secured a warrant that specified the seizure of any box that contained a document with Eileen Young's name on it. Regardless, the agents took whatever they wanted.

JERRY McDEVITT: *Eileen was Cyril's public and private secretary, so they knew she would be crucial to the investigation. They also had a warrant to search Eileen's laptop and, unbelievably, they seized the laptop itself. It may or may not have contained evidence of a crime, but it did contain other things. Prosecutors could have looked through Eileen's personal files, including pictures of her children or grandchildren, and so on. They weren't conducting a proper search. They were on a "fishing expedition."*

As the trial approached, prosecutors had still failed to answer the simple question that Mark Rush posed at the outset of the case: What witnesses would they call to substantiate the infamous body-snatching charge? It seems that the prosecution was prepared to present several written agreements between me and Carlow officials that allowed me to work at the university, but nothing more. According to Jerry McDevitt, at that point, Mary Beth Buchanan "started flipping."

JERRY MCDEVITT: *She said, "We look forward to cross-examining the nun [who was then president of Carlow University]." Then I said, "Mary Beth, you've never been in a courtroom if you're looking forward to cross-examining a nun. To cross-examine a priest is one thing, but a nun? Are you kidding me?"*

My general (and well-founded) paranoia notwithstanding, I began to see a villain behind every tree. Steve Zappala. Brad Orsini. And Mary Beth Buchanan. Together, they were after my scalp.

TIM UHRICH: *We could go into the whole Shakespearean drama of the battle between Cyril and Steve Zappala but, after all, here's what we had: Cyril did some dumb things, management-wise. A lot of Cyril's problems had to do with his thinking that, when you are kind to people, they're going to be kind back. I'm talking now about some employees in his own office who turned on him.*

These people only added fuel to the pyre that Zappala, Orsini and Buchanan were preparing. What's interesting and not generally appreciated about Brad Orsini is the fact that he once commented that Pittsburgh was the most politically corrupt city in America, which is saying something given that he hailed from Newark, once the land of Sharpe James, one of the most corrupt mayors in American history.

I've lived most of my life in Pittsburgh and have had an inside look at its government and politics. And while it may be a lot of things, good and not-so-good, it is no more or less corrupt than any other city in America. I had been a student of such things, as both an insider and outsider, when it comes to the political maelstrom.

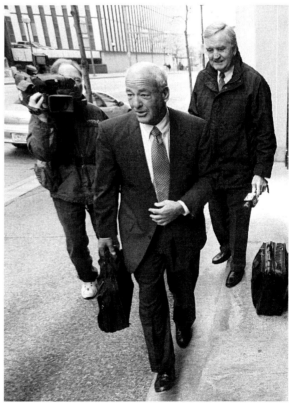

Heading to federal court in Pittsburgh, January 10, 2008 (*Associated Press*).

And for most of my life, I have distrusted those who wield power—locally and elsewhere—especially those involved in government. They're bastards, many of them. It's really unwise to turn your back to them. If you do, they will get you.

As I arrived in federal court on a characteristically overcast and blustery Pittsburgh morning in January 2008, I asked myself: "What have I done to deserve this?" I opened my mouth. That's what I did. I had to stand up for what was right and just.

"Be a doctor and
you will be your own boss"

My father never missed an opportunity to talk about me. He could be seen and heard from 8:00 a.m. until 11:30 p.m., seven days a week, greeting the patrons of his modest grocery store in Pittsburgh's "Lower Hill," and telling them all about his "Sonny." With cigar in hand, in his Yiddish-Lithuanian accent, my father told all who would listen about my bright future. He was determined that I would not be a shopkeeper like him.

Nathan Wecht, my father, and my mother, Fannie (née Rubinstein), immigrated to Western Pennsylvania in the tumultuous years surrounding the Russian Revolution, when violent pogroms drove many Jews to seek refuge in America. Dad hailed from Vilna (now called Vilnius), Lithuania, and Mom, from a small town near the city of Kyiv, in Ukraine.

My father was the middle of three children, with a younger sister and an older brother. His brother, David, remained in Lithuania, where he was murdered, along with six-million other Jews, in the Holocaust. For the most part, non–Jewish Lithuanians assisted the Nazis in their evil enterprise. My father's sister, Sarah, left Lithuania and made her way to "Eretz Yisrael" (Hebrew meaning "Land of Israel"), along with the re-markable Latvian Jew she married and with whom she later raised two sons, my Israeli cousins Yehuda and Ze'ev.

Dad made only one trip back to Lithuania to visit his parents, in 1937. The situation there, particularly for Jews, was already dire. He never had enough money or influence to bring his parents to America, and I don't know if they would have come if he had. But I'll tell you this: His mother's name was on his lips when he died.

My mother hailed from a much larger family. She had two brothers and four sisters. All of the Rubinstein girls were destined to become homemakers and helpers to their husbands, and all emigrated to America to begin new lives. My mother's father had been murdered on a train by anti–Semitic, Ukrainian thugs. Her mother and brothers remained in Ukraine and later perished in the Holocaust, after the Wehrmacht leveled the western areas of the Soviet Union. Sadly, all five of the Rubinstein girls ended up with breast cancer, and my mother was the last of them to die from it. I guess they carried that particular gene which has been talked about so much in recent years and, therefore, were predisposed to the disease.

As a young man, Dad studied the Talmud, the scholarly commentaries on the Bible that form the basis of much Jewish law, and he maintained his interest in the traditions of learning all his life. Unfortunately, as poor Jews in Eastern Europe, Mom and Dad had been denied the opportunity to acquire much formal education. Maybe that's why I was always driven to pursue advanced learning for myself. But my parents were both bright people, and I don't say that just because I was their son. They met in the United States, got married in Pittsburgh and, thereafter, did what many immigrants did and still do: They set up shop to sell things. In the case of my parents, those things were foodstuffs.

Mom and Dad established their first grocery store in Bobtown, a gritty, coal-mining hamlet founded by the Shannopin Coal Company in the 1920s. The little town hugs a small mountainside in Greene County, Pennsylvania, close to the West Virginia border. Theirs was a simple shop, offering staples for coal miners and their families.

Life was lean in the throes of the Great Depression, but before long, my parents were blessed (which is what they always told me). On March 20, 1931, my mother gave birth to a son who would ultimately be her only child. So began my life. For my first year, Mom and Dad did their best to make it in Bobtown. But faced with the hardships of the Depression, they decided to move to the "big city," to be closer to friends. Our first stop was McKees Rocks, a borough on Pittsburgh's western border. There they again set up shop. Dad ran the store with help from Mom, who also shouldered responsibility for the housework, and my childhood needs.

Life improved slowly and, after six years of hard work, my parents chose to move their business yet again, this time to Pittsburgh's Lower Hill District, to the corner of Marion and Locust streets. There, on the ground floor of a modest, rented building, they set up shop for what would be the last time, as I started third grade at Forbes Elementary School. Through all the moves and changes, one thing remained constant: For my parents, raising me was their primary purpose.

ARTHUR GROSSMAN: *Cyril's father was a grocer who struggled to make a living in hard times, and his parents always pushed him to be the best. He was their only child and they wanted nothing but success for him, and Cyril was determined to please them.*

As devoted as they were to me, Mom and Dad were also dedicated to "Wecht's Grocery." I remember the ever-present cleaver, and Mom and Dad cutting steaks

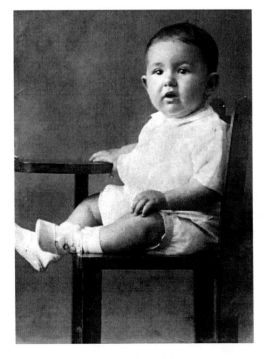

Cyril Harrison Wecht, age 1.

and chops themselves. They ran a more complete store this time around, albeit small, including candy, ice cream, produce, and freshly cut meats.

As a kid, I remember going with my father to the Strip District and seeing the trains pull up to unload produce, eggs, and so on. We also went to meat-packing places in and around Pittsburgh, and there were some big ones at the time, such as Armour & Company, and Oswald & Hess. It was pretty dramatic to see, at such a young age, animals being slaughtered and butchered. For the sake of a good story, I'd like to say that those experiences with death influenced and prepared me for what was to come in my career many years later. But that would be total bullshit. Nothing like that ever entered my mind.

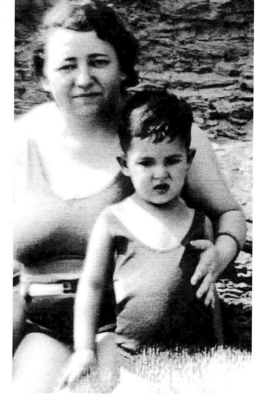

Age 3, with my mother, Fannie Rubinstein Wecht.

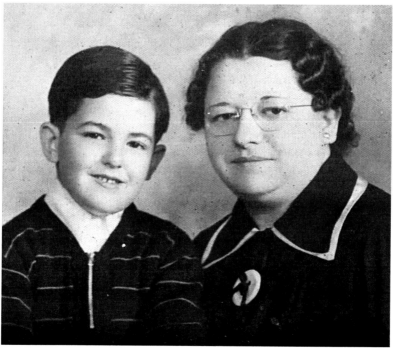

Age 5, with my mom.

At home, Mom maintained a tiny but functional kitchen and was a marvelous cook, especially with "old country" Jewish food. She had a quick mind and learned great recipes as well from all the wonderful Italian women who lived in the neighborhood. The quality of cuisine in the Wecht home was not lost on me, I assure you. But as for my father, he would have eaten flank steak and potatoes seven days a week, if given the choice.

Work days were long, but my parents labored together to make the store a modest success, with an occasional hand from neighborhood women who helped mind me during store hours. And as I grew, my dad, the shopkeeper, made it a point to extol the virtues of the medical profession. "Be a doctor and you will be your own boss," he would say. For my father, and indeed for many first-generation Jews in America, being a physician was the best thing one could be and, from the outset, he told me that I simply must become one. I was an obedient child, so I never questioned this. Looking back, I suppose that my eventual success was my father's success, too. I think he lived vicariously through me.

SAM SHAPIRO: *Cyril's father was a driving personality. He was like Cyril, except unsophisticated. Nathan Wecht was a shopkeeper, essentially, and where will that track take you? Maybe you make a few bucks. But Cyril got onto the right track, which was to go to college and become a professional. Nathan made sure that he got on a track that would take him somewhere.*

By all accounts, my parents kept a close eye on me. After all, for me to become a doctor, as planned, I had to be kept off the streets and out of trouble. Unlike the children of many of our neighbors, there would be no playing "craps"—maybe a little pinochle and bowling would be acceptable—and no shooting pool. One time, my father caught me coming out of the neighborhood pool hall, and was very distressed. I promised not to do it again but, nonetheless, I continued to sneak in from time to time.

To help keep me on the straight-and-narrow, at age seven, my parents started me on the violin. In no time, I was taking four lessons a week. Dad would drive me to my teacher or, if the weather was bad, I took a street car from our home to Murray Avenue in Squirrel Hill, and climbed the stairs to the second floor, above what was then the Waldorf Bakery, for my lessons.

At that time, Tuesday and Thursday nights, and Saturday and Sunday mornings for me were all about the violin—

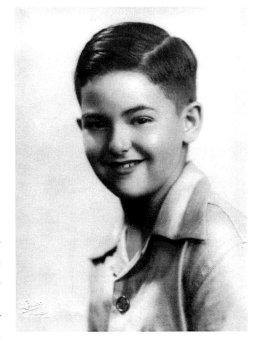

Age 7.

and discipline. In addition to the lessons, I was expected to practice four hours per day Monday through Friday, and six hours each on Saturday and Sunday. In time, I became very skilled and could play, from memory, some of the great violin concertos of Beethoven, Brahms, Mendelssohn and Tchaikovsky, and all five movements of Lalo's *Symphonie Espagnole.*

When I was 14, I began performing occasionally for local groups and organizations, such as the Young Men and Women's Hebrew Association (YM&WHA), which had a beautiful concert hall where major artists played from time to time. I also played at Carnegie Music Hall in Oakland, and was named to the Pittsburgh Youth Symphony Orchestra, the latter during my senior year of high school. I was good, but I didn't take to it of my own volition. I did it because my father made me. But as I got better at it, I did derive some pleasure from it.

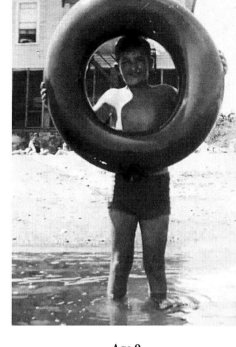

Age 9.

FRANCIS SHINE: *Some kids would go down after school and listen to Cyril play violin in the rear of his parents' store. In school and as a person, he was many things rolled into one. He was a musician, a brain, and an athlete. He was good at everything. And I don't know if he ever slept. He wouldn't do anything half-assed, not even if he was scrubbing the floor of his parents' store.*

Pittsburgh's Hill District was divided in half by Fifth Avenue, the demarcation between the Upper Hill and Lower Hill. On the upper side, it was predominantly black. On the lower side, it was Irish, Italian and Slavic, with a few Scots and others thrown in for good measure. A few Jewish families lived there, too. The neighborhood was lower middle-class, given that a large percentage of the community was comprised of first-generation immigrants, and many of the children were sent to religious schools, particularly Catholic ones. And like me, most of them went on to Fifth Avenue High School.

Then as always, I was a busy person who never wanted to miss out on anything. When I entered Fifth Avenue High in the fall of 1943, the school's music director had already heard about my violin skills and named me concertmaster of the student orchestra. In addition to this position, I was elected president of my class every year and, ultimately, became valedictorian at graduation. I also played baseball, basketball, and football.

HOP KENDRICK: *We always knew when Cyril was around. He was a football player, but maybe a bit limited, from our point-of-view. One day, when he was playing fullback and fumbled the ball, we called out to him—as a joke, of course—"You see, Wecht, I told you Jews can't play football." Cyril got pretty hot about that. On the next play, Nathan and Fannie Wecht's pride and joy, fueled by our perceived insult, purposely tipped the ball over the fence and it rolled down to the highway. Footballs were hard to come by in those days, and because of our teasing, and Cyril's volatile temper, there would be no football in the Lower Hill for a while.*

All through my youth in the Hill District, I was good friends with most of my neighbors, including the African Americans. We got into it once in a while, but we never had what I would call a "racial incident." We were all poor and had to struggle to be recognized. Sure, there was some fighting, but no drugs, at least none that I ever saw. Having witnessed, time and again, flashes of the temper that would, over time, come to characterize my public persona at least, Hop Kendrick developed his own theory about the genesis of my pugnacious nature, and he might be correct.

HOP KENDRICK: *In Nazi Germany, Jews were often portrayed as being docile. They stood near the ditches they had dug for themselves and didn't try to run, didn't try to defend themselves, and they were killed. This was totally unthinkable to Cyril. I don't know if this is true or not, but I have often thought that Cyril, consciously or unconsciously, vowed to himself never to go down without a fight, no matter what the situation. And I have always respected him for that.*

During my time as an adolescent, The Hill was one of America's most vibrant ethnic neighborhoods. Often called "Little Harlem," because of the large number of African Americans who lived there, it was a bustling place and home to a music scene that few cities could match. Jazz was the music of choice then, and the nightlife scene, including great haunts such as the famed Crawford Grill, and the Bamboola and Loendi clubs, made it a great place to hang out.

On any given Sunday, the neighborhood would be treated to a softball game between its Irish and Italian contingents. Sometimes the games were good-natured; sometimes not. But being Jewish in that melting pot of a community, I felt a sense of "otherness," which bothered me. If the Slavs, for example, were trying to put together a team for something, we hoped that they wouldn't have enough of their own because, if they didn't, they wouldn't object to Jews playing.

Now, I'm not telling you that there weren't any blatantly anti–Semitic sentiments in my day. In fact, once, when I was very young and we were still living in McKees Rocks, my mother was giving me a bath and I asked her, "Did I kill someone named Jesus?" She inquired as to why I would ask such a question. I told her, "Because someone said that I did." And when we moved to the Lower Hill, I remember some vicious anti–Semitic comments, though that tapered off after a few years.

When I was still just a small child, one of my mother's sisters, who lived in Pittsburgh, met a young Jewish man from New Haven, Connecticut. He was a student at the University of Pittsburgh School of Dentistry and, in my estimation, a pretty upstanding guy. The couple got married and moved to New Haven and, in the summertime, they rented a small cottage in Woodmont, Connecticut, the beach area between Milford and New Haven, on Long Island Sound. When I was two years old, my mother, during her time off from the store in the summer, began taking me to Woodmont to visit her sister. I remember traveling there by train, and will never forget the presence of soldiers, and the struggles to get a seat. Once there, we would stay in a little cottage at the beach, where I came to love the sun and, over the years, I made good friends.

Woodmont is about 90 minutes from New York City, 20 minutes from Bridgeport, and only 15 minutes from New Haven, the last of which I always thought of as my second home. My very closest friends were from there: Stuart Grodd, who ended up running one of the largest roofing companies in all of New England; and Murray Lender, whose immigrant father started to make bagels in his garage and grew the business into the world-renowned "Lender's Bagels."

By the time I was 15, my time in Woodmont began to pay dividends. I was spending entire summers there, during which I learned to be on my own. The young people there dated, had use of their fathers' cars, and even belonged to high school fraternities. It was a whole new social construct for me, and I could do this only because my father allowed it.

Back home, as a young teenager, on Saturday nights, I often went with my father to a bathhouse in the Upper Hill after closing the store at 11:30 p.m. We would stay at the "shvitz" for a few hours and then drive home in the middle of the night. I remember how bitterly cold it was in the winter. And the Upper Hill was a rough neighborhood at that time. Some of the local kids ended up in the penitentiary, a couple of them for murder. Others, ironically enough, became cops.

I think it's important here to clarify that, while I was an only child, I was never troubled by it. I never wished that I had siblings. I had many friends and was never starved for companionship. I never felt lonely. The Hill District was our world. None of us sat around thinking about how poor and unlucky we were. We didn't have, we didn't know, and we didn't care. We just lived our lives.

Typical of teenage boys in any era, my friends and I had our own rites of passage, one of which was to sneak into the Allegheny County Coroner's Office to view any dead bodies that might be on display in the refrigerated areas. Sometimes, the bodies lay on gurneys waiting to be viewed for purposes of identification by friends and family, or for pick-up by local funeral directors. The doors were always open and the deputy was usually sleeping in the back or busy in the lobby, so we would slip in on a dare to the large area just beyond, which was called "The Chapel," because of its stained-glass windows. I must admit that it was a little frightening because some of the fresher bodies were still dripping blood. What an interesting thing it would be for me to say that I first got interested in forensic pathology because of those daring youthful runs at the County Morgue. But like the negligible impact of my experiences in local slaughterhouses and meat packing plants as a little kid, this wouldn't be true either.

Another of our male-bonding experiences in those days was the river swim. Before the Parkway East was built, my buddies and I would travel on foot over the Boulevard of the Allies, and climb down to Second Avenue, then on to the Monongahela River. The steepness of the hillside made the trek treacherous. The first time I went, I was with older boys, and must admit to being scared shitless. In fact, I can remember at least one kid falling and being fatally injured. Several others were seriously hurt as well.

Nonetheless, we boys from The Hill accepted the risk, climbed down and swam in the river. I was a decent swimmer and, at that time, while the Monongahela River wasn't quite as filthy as the Ganges, it was close. Forget biological hazards. With the mills booming the way they were, producing the steel that helped us win the War, the industrial threat was far greater. But that's what kids did before television, video games, and the Internet. During the War, life wasn't so bad. I remember the "Victory Gardens," the curfews, and so forth. I can't tell you that none of us felt sorry for ourselves, but I sure didn't. My friends and I were happy just playing ball in the street.

Although my parents were poor and maybe under-educated, they weren't backward people. Mom and Dad were perennial subscribers to the Pittsburgh Symphony, and I accompanied my father, who loved classical music, to concerts on many a Sunday afternoon. My mother took me to plays and, as a kid, I remember seeing the great Paul Robeson, with his deep and booming voice, in *Othello*. I also liked movies and, luckily for me, the Rialto Theater was located just two blocks from our home. I took in serials there on Saturdays and cowboy fare on Sundays, not to mention the occasional musical.

In my day, we had amusements, but there was not much social life in the way that kids know it today, for better or worse. By the time I was a junior in high school, however, I would go with the other Jewish boys to the YM&WHA on Sunday nights. Nobody dated. Just kissing a girl was a big thing. My first formal date—in the sense that I called a girl and picked her up—was my high school prom.

In time, Italian families began to leave The Hill, to Brookline and Dormont; the Jews, to Oakland, East Liberty and Squirrel Hill; African Americans started moving out to Homewood-Brushton; and the Irish scattered to Greenfield and some to Oakland as well. No one made anybody relocate, but people tended to go with their own kind.

In the waning days of my high school experience, I had my eyes set on attending the University of Pittsburgh, but I learned, at the time, that my high school's principal had told Pitt's scholarship committee to beware of me because I was a "communist." After reading about the demise of the Nazis and the rise of the Soviet Union, I began discussing some of this with other kids at school. When the principal caught wind of this, he thought it was his duty to thwart the "Red Menace" at all costs. But I received a scholarship anyway, much to his chagrin, I'm sure.

In 1948, I was accepted at Pitt and there, as in high school, I became concertmaster of the orchestra. I also became an assistant to my violin teacher, Melitta Barjansky, who had become ill with a heart condition. I would help her and, in return, she would pay me a few dollars. To put it mildly, between my studies and my campus activities, including music, I led a whirlwind existence. And all of this was acceptable to my father because I was a registered college student, and in "pre-med," as planned.

During my college days, to save a buck or two, I lived at home with my parents

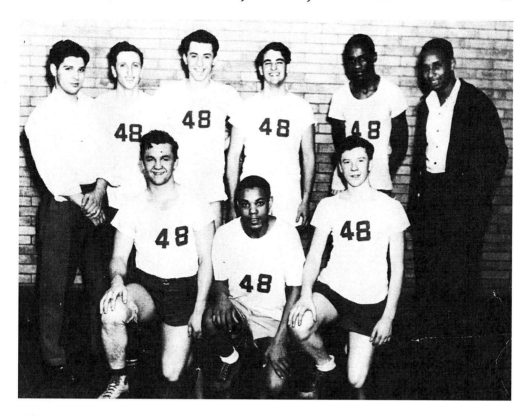

Fifth Avenue High School varsity basketball team, 1948. I am in the back row, fourth from the left.

in the Lower Hill. After all, it was a short commute to the university from there, and Mom's home cooking beat anything that I could get on campus. But in the spring of 1951, during my junior year, my parents, for the first time, purchased a home in the leafy-green Jewish enclave of Squirrel Hill, and I moved there with them. Things were getting better for my family, and it was a great time to be alive.

My good friend Sam Shapiro first met me when we became fraternity brothers at the then all–Jewish Phi Epsilon Pi at Pitt.

SAM SHAPIRO: *Cyril was ambitious, talented and always a leader. I related to him on many levels, including one important one: being Jewish. It was a burden for us to carry. When you're the first born of foreign parents, and your mother and father speak broken English—and you're Jewish on top of it all—there is something deep inside that makes you feel that you have to prove that you're as good as anybody else. Being Jewish drove Cyril toward achievement like no other factor in his life.*

During my time at Pitt, some people described me as a BMOC: a "Big Man on Campus." I was president of the student body and my fraternity; concertmaster of the orchestra; business manager of the campus newspaper and of the "Pitt Players" theater group (for which I also played the lead role in the school's production of Thornton Wilder's *Our Town*). And I was a varsity debater. I was president of everything, even of the university YMCA—as a Jew!

At Pitt, I was a good student and graduated with honors. It would have taken four people to accomplish what I did while I was a student there. But I wasn't selected as the outstanding senior. To this day, it's impossible for me to understand.

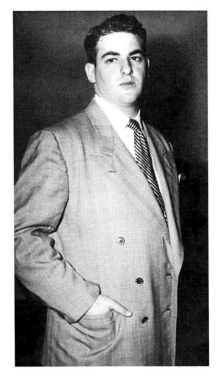

SAM SHAPIRO: *The one thing I know that Cyril wanted but did not accomplish at Pitt was having his name inscribed on the ODK walk, an honor bestowed every year to the outstanding senior man at the university by the national leadership honor society Omicron Delta Kappa. Cyril deserved that honor but didn't get it, and I think it was because certain people didn't like him.*

Speak with anyone about me and they'll talk about my temper, which I have never been afraid to use, sometimes to my benefit; sometimes not. My "in-your-face" personality has helped me throughout my life to achieve many things. I was then and still am aggressive. But my short fuse has also resulted in me having to pay, sometimes, a steep price.

"Big man on campus." At the University of Pittsburgh, 1951.

SAM SHAPIRO: *Cyril was the kind of person who said what he thought and, at times, didn't stop to think, "Might this hurt me?" He was outspoken, direct and articulate. But it's one thing to tell someone something they don't want to hear, and another to look someone in the eye and say, "You're an asshole," which is kind of what he did, sometimes.*

In my junior and senior years, I had little time for class as I bounced around campus, trying to run the university. Nonetheless, I received my B.S. in the spring of 1952 and, that fall, headed off to medical school.

Pitt may not like to admit it but, in those days, the university's medical school had a fixed quota of no more than 100 new students per year, of which no more than 10 could be Jew-

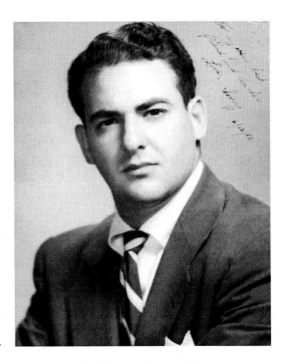

College graduate, 1952.

ish. This policy reduced the odds of my acceptance but, I still say that there was another more personal reason why I was not accepted to med school at my alma mater.

During my senior year at Pitt, as student body president, I was quoted in the *Pitt News* wondering innocently why there had never been an African American player on the school's basketball team. Reading what I had said, head basketball coach H.C. "Doc" Carlson, who was a major figure at Pitt's Department of Athletics and had lots of connections, went insane. He stormed into the student congress meeting with a copy of the offending issue in hand and carried on like a madman. I knew that Carlson had a dental degree from Pitt and I still believe that, because of my perceived impudence, he did whatever he could to make sure that I wasn't accepted into med school at the university. So, I headed off to the University of Buffalo School of Medicine, in New York, which was an odd place for a dyed-in-the-wool Pittsburgher.

Indeed, those were not easy times for Jews or blacks in America. And I'm not going to bullshit anyone and say that these things didn't bother me, that I'm above it all. You bet your ass they bothered me a lot then, and they still bother me today. But by 1955, Doc Carlson was gone from Pitt, and Julius Pegues became the school's first African American basketball player.

For my third year of medical school, I was able to transfer from Buffalo to Pitt, which pleased not only me but my parents as well. That year, I bought my first car. It wasn't much, but it was mine. I had gained my license at 16, but never drove Dad's old station-wagon, which he used primarily for chores and runs for the store. By the time I arrived back at Pitt, I had been thinking, on-and-off for at least a year, about something

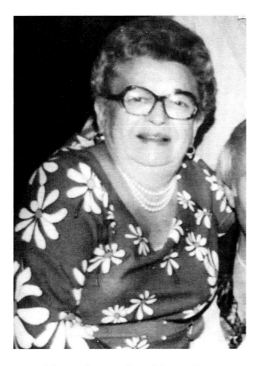

My mother, and my biggest fan.

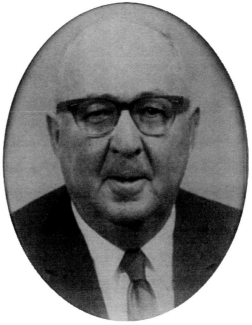

Nathan Wecht, my father, as he was known and loved.

called "legal medicine." I don't know what first brought it to mind, the idea of becoming a doctor *and* a lawyer. I never really reached a point where I thought about doing anything other than just going to medical school. But while wearing both professional hats intrigued me, I was definitely conflicted about it.

A natural born letter-writer—a skill and tendency that, for my entire life, has showcased my better side in notes of congratulations and thanks to family, friends and colleagues, and my worst in critical and vitriolic missives to my detractors—I wrote to the American Medical Association (AMA) for information about becoming a "double-threat," so to speak, in the nation's two most esteemed professions. As it turned out, my timing couldn't have been better.

In 1955, the AMA and the American Bar Association (ABA) were teaming up to present their first Biennial Medical-Legal Symposium in New York City. The AMA put me in touch with a man named Louis Regan, who was a doctor and lawyer from the West Coast and, at that time, one of the major figures in the field of legal medicine. Dr. Regan was to be the symposium's keynote speaker. He responded graciously to a letter I sent to him, and invited me to attend the symposium free of charge. So, I drove to New York with a nurse I was dating at the time, for a nice, however short, weekend. Dr. Regan spent 15 or 20 minutes with me while everybody was waiting to speak with him, and gave me some perspective on his field of work. From that moment on, my mind was made up. I was going into legal medicine.

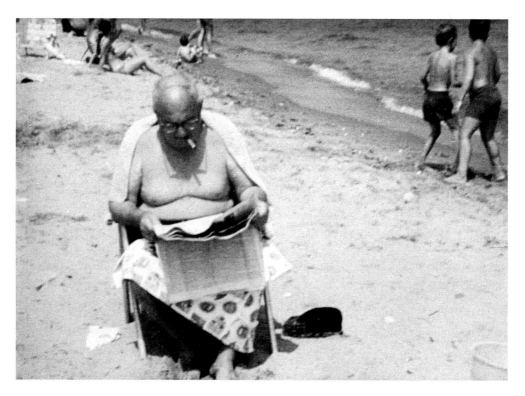

Like me, my father enjoyed the sun, and the news.

Love and Early Skirmishes

My interest in becoming both a doctor and a lawyer remained strong and led me to make further inquiries regarding the efficacy of doing so. I came to learn that pathology—forensic pathology, in particular—was the most integrated medical field insofar as legal applications were concerned. So, after a required, year-long rotating medical internship, I applied to law school. I chose Pitt because I had already been admitted to the pathology residency program at the Veterans Administration hospital located in the Oakland section of Pittsburgh, not far from my home.

Fortunately for me, Dr. Edwin R. Fisher, an outstanding pathologist in his own right and a professor in the Department of Pathology at Pitt, gave me permission to attend law school during my residency, as long as I fulfilled my obligations on the pathology side. So, there I was, a full-time law student—getting grades good enough to make law review—and a full-time medical resident in pathology. What's more, as a resident, between 1957 and 1959, I averaged three overnight shifts per week, plus a 24-hour shift on two of every three weekends, while also covering emergency rooms and in-house medical services at three hospitals: South Side, Homestead, and Suburban General.

During my time as a pathology resident, an organization called the Allegheny County Medical Society formed what was known as the Committee for the Medical Examiner System. The Society's Chairman, Dr. Ralph J. Stalter, an internist, and I had met several years earlier, during my third and fourth years of med school, when I served as a junior intern at Pittsburgh's St. Francis Hospital. Dr. Stalter knew that I was attending law school and wanted to become a forensic pathologist, so he offered me a seat on the new committee.

With the aid of my fellow committee members, I began to compile information about new developments in forensic pathology, while examining the inner workings of the Allegheny County Coroner's Office, which we found incredibly backward, and said so—publicly. In those days, at approximately 1.65 million, Allegheny County's population was somewhat larger than it is today. But we were the most backward large metropolitan area in the country when it came to medical-legal investigation. Nonetheless, as I approached my final year of law studies, life threw me a curveball. I was called upon to prepare for military service under the auspices of the "Berry Plan."

Named after Frank B. Berry, M.D. (who had served in both world wars and rose, in 1954, to become Assistant Secretary of Defense for Health and Medical Affairs), the plan allowed for medical students to finish school and complete their residencies and specialties before being called for military service. Instead of grabbing everyone when they graduated and ending up with a bunch of general practitioners, they waited for us to become specialists—surgeons, pathologists, and so forth. My aspirations as a law student were of no concern to them, but at least I was deferred from serving for two years, which they figured would be enough time for me to become a pathologist. When I finished my second year of residency, in 1959, I headed off to serve in the United States Air Force.

As a man in uniform, I caught a break by being stationed at the Air Force's largest hospital, Maxwell Air Force Base, in Montgomery, Alabama. Comprising more than 400 beds and staffed with specialists in a variety of medical fields, it was the Air Force's hub when it came to pathology. Approximately 28 Air Force bases throughout the Southeast regularly sent us specimens for study, and the workload kept me and my military colleagues plenty busy—yet, typically, not busy enough for me. But before long, the full-court press of my professional life and personal ambition was tamed ever so slightly by a young and attractive Norwegian-born woman: Sigrid Ronsdal, Airman Third Class.

SIGRID WECHT: *I met Cyril in 1960, and wasn't all that attracted to him, at first. Actually, I was a bit frightened because, out of the blue, I got a call to report to "Captain Wecht" at the base hospital. "Am I in trouble?" I wondered. Well, I found out that Captain Wecht worked in the hospital pathology department, and was single, so I reported in as*

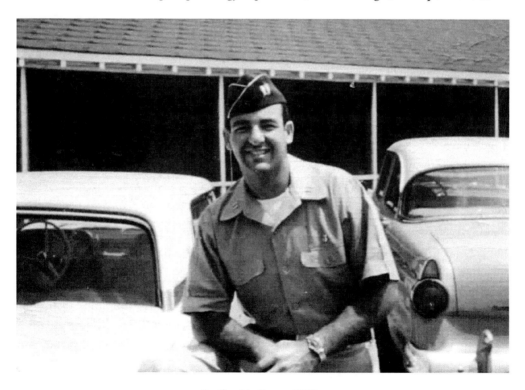

In the Air Force, 1959.

requested. Somehow, he knew that I was from Norway and said that he wanted me to meet the wife of a friend of his, who was Danish. I figured that he was asking me out on a double-date, and I said, "Sure."

Sigrid, who was about eight years younger than me, was a beautiful young lady who was raised on the outskirts of Oslo, Norway, in a nice house with an apple orchard.

Aside from World War II, and troubles with my father, I enjoyed my childhood very much. I loved being outdoors. Like most Norwegians, I liked skiing and hiking, and still have dreams of maybe going back someday to hike in the mountains another time or two.

But with the War raging in Europe, and a father who could be a scary person when provoked, Sigrid's childhood left something to be desired. She made it through, however, thanks to the strength of her mother.

Like Cyril, I was an only child. But unlike him, I was the child of an unhappy marriage, and my mother and I were yearning for a better life. My mother's family never came over to America, but she traveled back and forth between Norway and the United States with me several times, trying to escape my father, which is why we eventually ended up here.

In those days, for a woman to divorce, as Sigrid's mother had, was considered a shameful thing.

We left Norway for America in 1947, when I was eight years old, for a year initially. Thereafter, I saw my father very little. He was the gym director on a cruise ship that traveled to and from Norway and the U.S. Every time he came to America, he looked for us. At one point, we moved back to Norway, and my father found us there, too. Eventually, we were able to elude him permanently, and thank God for that.

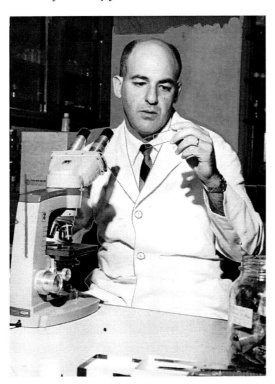

A career is born, 1960 (*Pittsburgh Post-Gazette*).

At the base in Montgomery, through the grapevine, I learned that the city's two hospitals each maintained its own pathologist. I also learned that these two pathologists despised one another. When one went on vacation or got sick, the other would refuse to cover, so I thought, "Why don't I cover for both of them?" My chief said, "Fine, but do it on your own time."

For two years, at the end of long work days, and even on weekends, I left the base and went in to read-out surgical specimens for whichever hospital I was covering. On top of that, I conducted autopsies, the facility for which was located in the local African American community. To enter, I had to walk, first, through a saloon and then a barbershop, before finally arriving at the "morgue," which was equipped with little more than a marble table. But in the end, I got credit for a third and fourth year of pathology training while doing my two years of military duty. With my medical training and military service finally under my belt, in 1961, I turned my attention toward completing a fellowship in forensic pathology and, hopefully, finishing the last year of my law studies. "With that fellowship and a J.D.," I thought, "I'll be on my way."

I did some research and discovered an excellent forensic pathology program in the Medical Examiner's Office in Baltimore, Maryland. And through a cousin of mine, I became aware that the University of Maryland had a fine law school with a fully accredited evening division. So, after an honorable discharge from the Air Force, I went to Baltimore and finished my third year of law training in the evenings—carrying a full course-load—while, by day, I worked toward completing my fellowship in forensic pathology. In addition, I provided pathology services to a small Baltimore hospital. Sure, I was working my ass off, but I looked at life like this: Some things are handed to you; others are lucky breaks; and the rest is just hard work. Not many people could have done what I did, and I still can't explain how I covered so much ground in so little time.

SIGRID WECHT: *Cyril left the Air Force and Montgomery to go to Baltimore and, luckily, I was able to get a transfer to Andrews Air Force Base in Washington, D.C. I lived with my mother, who happened to be in Baltimore at the time, and commuted from her apartment to the base every day while Cyril was going to law school and completing his fellowship. In time, we managed to get a "hardship discharge" for me by claiming that my mother was seriously ill. In Baltimore, I also started taking lessons to convert to Judaism, which Cyril wanted. On top of all that, we were planning to get married. It all happened very fast, like everything in America.*

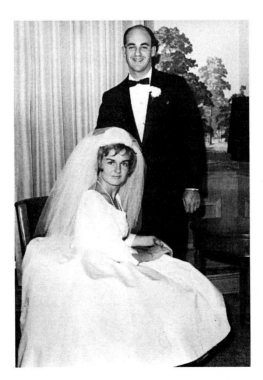

Sigrid and I on our wedding day, October 1961.

While still in Baltimore, Sigrid and I dashed off to Pittsburgh for a weekend to get hitched, and were married on Sunday, October 21, at Temple Rodef Shalom, which still stands proudly on the border between Oakland and Shadyside. Both of us had to be back at work on Monday morning, so we thought we'd hit the road after our nuptials and begin our life as newlyweds at Bedford Springs resort, which was on the way to Baltimore. Unfortunately, we blew a tire on the Pennsylvania Turnpike and had no choice but to skip our honeymoon and head home. Sigrid became a U.S. citizen and, not long after, Jewish, too.

SIGRID WECHT: *I was brought up in a Christian home, I guess, but I was always interested in other religions, and so was my mother. I thought, "What's the big deal? If you step back as a Christian far enough into history, you'll fall right into Judaism," which has a wonderful tradition. Little by little, I got used to the religion, the culture, and the food, and found it very appealing.*

After completing my fellowship in forensic pathology and collecting my law degree from the University of Maryland, Sigrid and I left Baltimore for good in the summer of 1962 and returned to my doting parents, and the city I would forever call my home.

SIGRID WECHT: *Cyril never considered going anywhere except back to Pittsburgh, to his parents. In fact, we lived with them for the first year of our marriage, during which time I had a baby, and was expecting another. My mother-in-law and father-in-law hovered over and cared for us. It was so wonderful. From them, I learned a lot about what being a family means.*

JUNE SCHULBERG: *Sigrid has always been Cyril's greatest advocate. He's a lucky guy to have found her. She's a strong and interesting woman in her own right. How many women do you know who, after raising four kids, would go to law school and become a lawyer?*

As the 20th century trudged past its midpoint, when it came to the performance of autopsies and the pursuit of forensic science endeavors, many counties in the U.S. began to jettison the traditional position of coroner in favor of a new medical examiner system. The essential difference between the two? Coroners are elected representatives of the people; medical examiners are governmental appointees. Allegheny County, however, was not moved by the winds of change. And, unfortunately, in those days, there was no more primitive coroner's set-up anywhere than that which existed in our county. From 1940 to 1960, the Allegheny County Coroner was a dentist named William D. McClelland. He was a Democrat powerhouse, an opponent within the Democratic party of famed Pittsburgh Mayor David L. Lawrence. McClelland maintained his dental practice and discharged his duties as Coroner on the side, aided by a retired pathologist named Dr. Theodore Helmbold, who was in his 70s. Dr. Helmbold would do an occasional autopsy, essentially homicides, but not necessarily all of them.

In 1960, William McClelland was elected County Commissioner, and his Chief Deputy Coroner, Joseph B. Dobbs, from Lawrenceville, was in line to succeed him. For years, Dobbs had earned his living as a carpenter and then moved up politically, in time, becoming Chief Deputy Coroner of Allegheny County. He never went to college. He had attended no medical school. He had no scientific credentials whatsoever. But he had politics and tradition on his side.

In those days, if the Coroner died, resigned, or was kicked out of office, the Chief Deputy would become "Acting Coroner" until the governor appointed either him or someone else. In the end, the governor did appoint him, and Dobbs held the Coroner's position through 1966. The appointment of a carpenter to the position of

Coroner (replacing a dentist, no less) wasn't an act of ignorance. And it wasn't a matter of money, either. The fact is, at that time, nobody cared who was Coroner, here or anywhere else.

In 1962, I was back in Pittsburgh, and soon became active again on Dr. Ralph J. Stalter's Committee for the Medical Examiner's System. As before, my colleagues and I continued to hammer away at the presiding County Coroner, Joseph Dobbs, and the antiquated system employed in his office, which hadn't even a microscope back then. And our committee upped the ante when we adopted a new slogan: "You can get away with murder in Allegheny County."

Needless to say, the choice of words was not appreciated in the halls of local government, but it referred only to the Coroner's Office. I was a forensic pathologist, after all, and knew what a coroner's office was supposed to be and do. So, as a forensic pathologist who had trained in one of the top medical examiner's offices in the country, I felt it necessary to work for changes. But Eugene L. Coon, who was then head of the Pittsburgh police department's homicide division, took exception to our "get away with murder" theme, feeling that it reflected badly on him and his officers. I didn't appreciate it at the time, but I soon came to learn that Coon, who was then sucking-up to the local Democratic Party, had a personal—and political—agenda all his own.

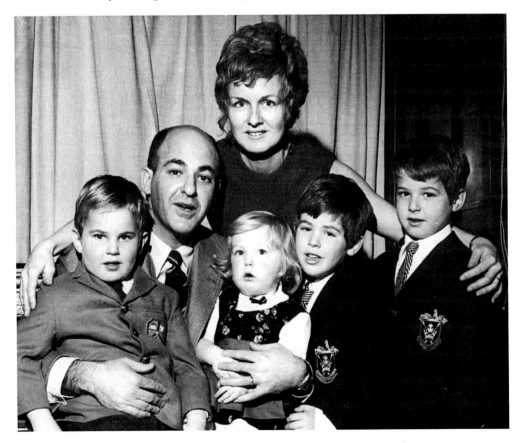

With Sigrid and our children: Ben, Ingrid, Daniel and David.

In 1964, when Robert W. Duggan, a Republican, upset the incumbent Democrat for district attorney, he reached out to me through an intermediary, a Republican attorney who had known me from our undergraduate days at Pitt. Duggan asked if I would consider being an assistant district attorney and his medical-legal advisor, and I answered in the affirmative.

Sophie Masloff, who graduated from Fifth Avenue High School years before me and was then an employee of the Allegheny Court of Common Pleas (and, eventually, Pittsburgh's first and only female Mayor, and first and only Jewish Mayor), remembers me from my days with Duggan.

SOPHIE MASLOFF: *I first met Cyril when he started working for Bob Duggan. He wasn't in the DA's office for more than a few days before he had the place in turmoil, and it never stopped. He fought with everyone. Duggan tolerated him, but Cyril didn't tolerate Duggan. In Pittsburgh, as in most cities, the DA worked closely with the police, and Cyril didn't like that. As a result, he and Duggan were constantly at odds.*

In November 1965, against an incumbent Democrat and with the full force of the Allegheny County Republican Party, Dr. William R. Hunt, a general surgeon from the nearby city of McKeesport, was elected Allegheny County Coroner, an eventuality that came about partially because of the ongoing barrage of criticism leveled by me and others against the previous Coroner and the state of his office. When Dr. Hunt took office in January 1966, I hopped aboard as his Chief Deputy Coroner and, in short order, he asked me to become his Chief Forensic Pathologist—a job I readily accepted. I then started to revise the office's approach and began to develop new scientific modalities. I ran everything very professionally, but still under horribly inadequate conditions.

By then, we finally had a microscope (an instrument that had been around since the end of the 16th century), albeit a basic one, but we still didn't have a proper autopsy table. Instead, we were using a cheap, mortuary-type table that one could find in the back of any funeral home, where embalming is done. But before long, we were able to purchase a brand-new porcelain autopsy table, and I went about designing and planning a whole new autopsy area.

At first, through the dead of that winter, I did all of the county's autopsies by myself in an unheated basement that was located just off the driveway in the back of the coroner's building. The driveway sloped downward into the garage, which is where bodies were brought in, after which they were taken away for autopsy. On the ground level was a crematorium (which continued to function for some years after we got there, until we closed it down) and a basement area that we used to store bodies. (Because of the smell, we did not like to bring them upstairs.) It was in that room that I did my work, with just a small floor heater for warmth. We set up our new table there and I performed autopsy after autopsy, freezing my ass off, wearing a tossle cap and a thick overcoat with an apron over it.

In February 1967, Dr. Hunt and I together attended the American Academy of Forensic Sciences meeting. While there, he received a phone call that would change both of our lives. It seems that the Allegheny County Republican Committee wanted him to run for County Commissioner. Dr. Hunt promptly left the meeting and, to make a long story short, returned to Pittsburgh, ran for County Commissioner, and was elected. So, on January 1, 1968, after just two years as Coroner, Dr. William R. Hunt had to step down to become one of three Allegheny County Commissioners. And his departure left two years of an unexpired four-year term available to some lucky appointee of the governor.

Everybody thought that I would be appointed, but Governor Raymond P. Shafer was a Republican and, to my disappointment, my old friend, Dr. Ralph J. Stalter, Chairman of the Medical Examiner's Committee, acquiesced to the prodding of his political allies and assumed the role of Coroner himself, with the proviso that he would simply fill out Dr. Hunt's term and then step aside to allow me to run for Coroner in 1969. Again, to my disappointment, when the time came, the Republicans pressured Dr. Stalter to run for reelection, and he did. But I ran against him, won, and assumed the role of Allegheny County Coroner on January 1, 1970.

As a doctor, lawyer and forensic scientist, I would go on to hold a variety of public offices in Allegheny County until as late as 2006. The question is: Why? Compared to the income potential of my private consulting business, Wecht Pathology Associates, which I founded in the late 1960s, the aforementioned positions would provide only modest remuneration, at best. So, the fact that I ran for public office could not have been motivated by money. But as time wore on and the demand for my services grew, I began functioning both inside and outside the county system.

JUNE SCHULBERG: *In addition to being Coroner, Cyril was a private medical-legal consultant. He would take cases from either criminal lawyers or plaintiffs' lawyers in civil cases where a medical-legal question was involved. He would gather all the records, write reports, and then meet and talk with the lawyers and, sometimes, even the parties or their surviving relatives. Many times, he would testify in court. That's one of the reasons he became so well known.*

But even after my election as Coroner, I still had no real political ambitions. Sure, I had opportunities to be a coroner or medical examiner in different places, but I chose to stay in Pittsburgh with my parents, wife, and kids, by which time I had four: three sons—David, Daniel and Benjamin—and one daughter, Ingrid. I was also becoming increasingly busy with medical-legal consultations in my private business. My involvement in politics came about only because of my involvement in Allegheny County as a forensic scientist.

When I took over as Coroner in 1970, a position for which I possessed more than the necessary credentials, I believed that I had finally arrived. "This is it, for me," I thought. Given my background, the Coroner's Office was where I belonged—that is until 1971, when Thomas J. Foerster and Leonard Staisey were up for reelection to the Allegheny County Board of Commissioners.

While acting as County Coroner, I had remained involved in the Democratic Party, and had a friendly relationship with Tom Foerster. But my old nemesis, Gene Coon, who still harbored antipathy toward me, had been elected Allegheny County

Sheriff in 1970, and became the county's Democratic Chairman in a fast shuffle behind the scenes.

The enmity that had developed years earlier between the two of us over the whole "get away with murder" campaign flourished and was fed upon by both of us as well as by each of our respective camps, becoming more heated as time went on. Soon, I found out that Coon was set to play a principal role in an attempted *coup d'état*. He and his cohorts were trying to engineer the removal of one of the incumbent County Commissioners. The way I saw it, Coon's plan was to maneuver Tom Foerster out of reelection by challenging and defeating him in the primary. Unfortunately for Gene Coon, I interceded. I backed Foerster and my efforts succeeded in pulling him through the Democratic primary in spring 1971—by a margin of less than 1,000 votes. I was reelected Coroner in 1973 and 1977 and, having served as a Democratic Committee member in my home district of Squirrel Hill, I decided to run for Chairman of the Allegheny County Democratic Committee—against none other than the ubiquitous Eugene Coon.

In 1978, I was in Washington, D.C., serving on the forensic pathology panel for the U.S. House of Representatives Select Committee on Assassinations, and was attending to this important job—reviewing and analyzing the Warren Commission Report regarding the assassination of President John F. Kennedy—when I received a phone call with news that I had vanquished the malevolent Gene Coon and won my bid to be the county's new Democratic Committee Chair—even though I hadn't been on the campaign trail for days. Then, toward the end of the year, I was approached by Tom Foerster with an idea. At that point, Tom was a minority County Commissioner, the lone Democrat serving alongside two Republicans on a three-person panel. So, he came to me and asked if I would run with him. I agreed to do so, and our bid was successful as we both won election in November 1979. I became a bona fide County Commissioner in January 1980.

I won't lie and say that, at that time, I still didn't have any interest in politics. But, truly, when Tom Foerster asked me to run for County Commissioner alongside him, I wasn't thinking about being anything other than being County Coroner. I was very busy in that role, and as a private medical-legal consultant. But it was no good denying the obvious any longer. Perhaps only as a by-product of my personal drive and professional ambition, I had indeed become "a politician."

By 1980, I had been elected Coroner three times, and County Commissioner to boot. I'd already served as President of the American College of Legal Medicine, and President of the American Academy of Forensic Sciences, and had been granted the opportunity to be the first non-governmental forensic scientist to review the autopsy materials of John F. Kennedy. One could say that I had reached the pinnacle of a productive career. But there was so much more to do.

Without question, my tenure as Allegheny County Coroner, like most of my professional endeavors, was not without controversy. While I was responsible for significant upgrades in professionalism and technology during my service from 1970 to 1980, which established the Allegheny County Coroner's Office as one of the best in the nation, my political activities proved problematic due to my shoot-from-the-hip style and unwillingness to run away from a fight.

Late in my tenure, I was accused of performing, at the County Morgue, autopsies for counties other than Allegheny, and depositing the fees for these services into the bank account of my private consulting firm. If true, such activities would surely have been a violation of the public trust. But this wasn't true, and it was none other than Gene Coon who stirred up all the trouble.

In January 1979, I picked up the local daily and read an article about me by Tom Snyder, the political courthouse reporter for *The Pittsburgh Press*. The piece was a sand-bag operation. Snyder never even called me to get my side of the story. In that article, all kinds of charges were leveled against me by Gene Coon, the most significant of them being that I, as County Coroner, had been doing private autopsies for my own personal gain. It was all bullshit. But Eugene Coon who, as noted, by then had risen to become County Sheriff, had it in for me. The story goes as follows.

When William R. Hunt was Allegheny County Coroner, he started something called the "Professional Education Fund" at the Coroner's Office. To his credit, Dr. Hunt reached out to coroners from other jurisdictions and said, "We'll do autopsies for you and charge you for them." Monies generated from the provision of these extra-county services were deposited into a fund that Dr. Hunt had established to be used to improve things in our office. When Dr. Hunt stepped down, Dr. Ralph J. Stalter continued what was called the Professional Education Fund during his tenure. We did the autopsies, and Dr. Charles Winek, who headed our forensic toxicology lab, did the testing.

The Professional Education Fund had existed for four years under two separate Coroners before me (both of whom were Republicans, by the way). I continued it, and it expanded greatly under me because of my growing reputation and the reputation of the office. Nonetheless, I was accused of doing this work illegally, and was eventually indicted on six state law counts—three felonies and three misdemeanors—based on allegations of financial misappropriation and the implication of a questionable relation-ship between my private and public offices.

In life, one must be lucky: Lucky in marriage; lucky with one's kids; lucky in one's choice of occupation, etc. And if a person finds him-or-herself with legal problems, he or she must be lucky in their choice of a lawyer, because one could inadvertently pick someone who may know the law, but is not a fighter. I had been lucky on all counts. Enter West Virginia's Stanley Preiser, an attorney whom I had come to know by work-ing with him on several cases. He believed in my innocence, and became my lawyer. Stanley was a skilled attorney: not a big-shot, but well-respected. And he was a fighter. He never developed the national reputation of some of the big-shot attorneys in the area, but all the big shots considered him as often better than they were.

In American jurisprudence, a preliminary hearing is a legal proceeding during which the prosecution presents its *prima facie* case, not beyond a reasonable doubt. The defendant cannot introduce evidence or bring witnesses. At the conclusion of the hear-ing, a judge or magistrate then decides whether or not the case has a logical, substantive and legitimate basis. At my preliminary hearing, the prosecution presented its strongest points and the judge dismissed one felony and one misdemeanor immediately. So, we went to trial with two felonies and two misdemeanors remaining.

The prosecution, under the direction of District Attorney Robert E. Colville, formerly the Chief of Police in Pittsburgh, presented a host of witnesses. He even brought in other forensic pathologists to dump on me; not to deal with the issues, but to assassinate my character. Given that most of the judges in town were friendly with me (I had worked with and helped many of them win their offices), the prosecution called on Stephen Zappala, Sr., a Justice on the Pennsylvania Supreme Court, and encouraged him to issue an edict saying, in effect, that no judge in Allegheny County was eligible to preside over my case, and that a judge would be appointed by the Supreme Court itself. Naturally, the Court appointed a Republican judge from Meadville, Pennsylvania. But there again, I got lucky. That judge turned out to be an honorable, decent person, and was eminently patient and fair.

After six weeks of the prosecution's case, in which my attorney Stanley Preiser did little more than cross-examine the government's witnesses, the specially-appointed Republican judge threw out one of the remaining felonies and one of the misdemeanors—and we hadn't even presented our first witness. The prosecution realized what was happening and became determined not to allow the jury to take the easy way out by coming in with a verdict of "guilty" on an insubstantial misdemeanor charge, while acquitting me on a felony. Hence, the prosecution moved to withdraw the remaining misdemeanor. We objected, but the judge said that the prosecution had a right to withdraw a charge, if they wished. At that point, all that was left was one felony charge, and the trial proceeded. In the end, the jury was out for only a few hours. The next day, they came in with an acquittal. The ordeal was over. That was in 1981. But there was a sequel.

Apparently, Gene Coon and others were still agitating behind the scenes, and were able to convince Allegheny County Controller Frank Lucchino to go after me civilly for monies that had been deposited in the Professional Education Fund and had been spent without the permission of the County Commissioners. Another hand-picked judge was appointed and, after a preliminary hearing with Judge Nicholas Papadakos, the county decided that they didn't like the way things were going and took the case away from him. In place of Papadakos, they assigned the case, in my estimation, to a blatantly partisan Republican judge named Albert E. Acker, who was from another county. And that's when we made a mistake.

I don't blame David Armstrong, my lawyer at the time, because we talked about the problem we faced and agreed on a solution. We decided to go "non-jury" because we felt that the facts were in our favor. We could show what the fund was and for what it was used. I wasn't in the room and didn't learn about this until later but, according to David Armstrong, Judge Acker said to him something to this effect: "I want you to know that Cyril Wecht is not going to get away with some of the same things he did when he testified before me the last time." David did not know this, but I had appeared several years earlier in Albert E. Acker's courtroom in a northern, rural Republican county, at the first medical malpractice case ever heard there in which there was a verdict for the plaintiff. A hot-shot attorney named Francis Shields, from Philadelphia, represented the doctor. I testified for the plaintiff and the jury came in with the proper verdict. So, what did I get away with? I succeeded in testifying, that's all.

If David Armstrong had told me then and there what Judge Acker had said to him, I don't know if we could have had him removed, but we sure as hell would have tried. In any case, Judge Acker heard my civil case and came down with a verdict that I call, at best, cockamamie. He recalculated the civil damages to the county and said that I owed in excess of $200,000.

Somewhat uncharacteristically, the Controller had been smart enough to say, before the civil trial was over, that my predecessors, Drs. Hunt and Stalter, also owed money to the county, albeit smaller amounts, because both held the Coroner's position for only two years each. But I had held the post for the better part of 10 years and processed many more cases than did either of my predecessors. Drs. Hunt and Stalter both capitulated and paid money, but I refused.

Although Judge Acker did say in his opinion that not one penny of the fund had gone to me for any private purpose, the court found that we had not received permission from the County Commissioners or the Controller to establish such a fund and solicit money. The court's contention was that the money should have gone to the county at large, and not to the Coroner's Office.

As Coroner, I was held responsible for this breach of protocol, even though the money was spent legitimately on new equipment and current reference books, to cover the expenses for doctors to attend professional meetings, and to reimburse transporta-

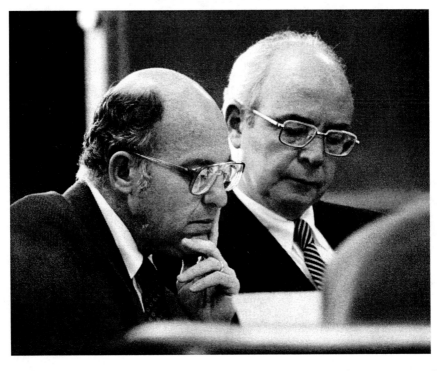

Allegheny County takes aim at me. My first public corruption trial, with attorney David Armstrong, 1980 (*Pittsburgh Post-Gazette*).

tion costs for prospective residents in forensic pathology to come in for interviews. All of this was documented, but we never sought permission. We didn't know that we had to do this. After holding out for a time, I agreed to settle with the county for roughly $170,000, and decided not to waste time on an appeal.

MARK SCHWARTZ: *After the trial in 1980, every politician wrote Cyril off. Everyone that he heretofore had been friends with, knifed him in the back. You're not talking about enlightened people with advanced degrees. You're talking about petty people who were very powerful.*

Anyway, having been elected County Commissioner in 1979, I was up for reelection in 1983. Admittedly, I had been badly weakened by the legal actions that had been brought against me, and this only fueled my opposition. As a result, the Democratic race became a free-for-all. In addition to Tom Foerster and I, the incumbents, Pittsburgh Mayor Pete Flaherty threw his hat in the ring, as did my arch nemesis, Eugene Coon. Would my political winning streak continue?

At a well-attended nomination endorsement meeting in February, the Democratic Committee rejected Tom Foerster and endorsed me for re-election. The committee then paired me, unbelievably, with Gene Coon. Foerster then teamed up with Pete Flaherty, and the two ran against Coon and me for the two Democratic nominations, and narrowly defeated us. It wasn't too big a deal. I went back to my private consulting. Coon continued on as County Sheriff. But it wouldn't be long until I flirted with politics again.

The Golden Rule
"He who has the gold, rules"

If you spoke with people who have been close to me, some might tell you that I was never well-suited to live and work in a small, provincial city such as Pittsburgh. Tim Uhrich, a former political campaign aide of mine and formerly Solicitor for the Allegheny County Coroner's Office during my tenure, has known me for a long time, both as a politician and as a forensic pathologist.

> TIM UHRICH: *Cyril is a Jewish liberal whose style is much better suited to the Upper West Side of Manhattan than it is to Pittsburgh. He was born and raised here, but he's not a "Pittsburgh-type guy," and that's one of the reasons why, politically, Cyril has had so many problems here.*

I don't agree with Tim on this. As the reader, feel free to make your own decision about it.

Tim Uhrich came to Pittsburgh in 1980 from Allentown, Pennsylvania, in the eastern part of the state, the year I finished my first 10-year stint as Coroner of Allegheny County.

> *Many Democrats here are just liberal Republicans. That's why Arlen Specter did so well in Western Pennsylvania. He was a moderate Republican; a Democrat in a finer suit.*

Tim's relocation to Pittsburgh was precipitated by a desire to finish his undergraduate studies. Up until that point, he had been a newspaper reporter for the *Allentown Morning Call*, an exhilarating job that had aced-out college for the young man's attention. He had also worked for the Mayor of Allentown. But at the age of 30, he enrolled at Pitt with the goal of getting into its law school. In any case, after two years of living here, Tim got wind of my public corruption trial, which was making headlines locally. Indeed, the Pittsburgh media had done a number on me.

> *What I knew about Cyril back then was only what I had read in newspapers and saw on TV, and the impression that I had was not good. By 1982, I had finished my undergraduate work and intended to go to law school, so I was not seeking employment. Unfortunately, I didn't make the cut for Pitt law, and needed something to do. So, it was timing that brought Cyril and me together.*

Not counting my public corruption trial, the early 1980s was a good time for me, and all devout Democrats in Pennsylvania, for that matter. The state hadn't yet started to trend Republican, which meant that it was still largely a Democratic stronghold, and incumbent Governor Richard Thornburgh, a Republican, appeared vulnerable. In the estimation of Tim Uhrich, and any number of other key Democrats in the region, Thornburgh's problem was that there weren't enough Republican-based races in the 1982 election cycle to guarantee a substantial Republican turnout.

TIM UHRICH: *The statewide Democratic Party was desperate to find someone credible to run against Dick Thornburgh. The Party was, in fact, looking for a "sacrificial lamb," and that role was perfect for Cyril, who was, at the time, serving as a County Commissioner in Allegheny County.*

Tim's recollection is that the Party wanted me to run for Governor but, at the very notion of that, I quipped, "That's roads, bridges, sewers, and that kind of stuff, right?" In other words, I had no interest in the job but, rather, had my sights set on a much bigger prize—the U.S. Senate. A perch atop Capitol Hill would afford me the opportunity to debate the pressing issues of the day, such as what was going on in the Middle East, and the challenges facing the national economy.

That's what was driving him. And lo and behold, a man named Allen Ertel came to the rescue, agreeing (perhaps as the aforementioned "lamb to the slaughter") to do battle with Dick Thornburgh as Pennsylvania's Democratic gubernatorial candidate. So, Cyril was off the hook. Ertel was the former DA in Lycoming County and a U.S. Congressman but, quite frankly, a "nothing" as a candidate. He had no charisma and did not connect with people, yet he came within only 100,000 votes of unseating Thornburgh.

Had I decided to run, with my boundless energy and what Tim calls my "raw magnetism," I might well have become Governor of Pennsylvania. But I knew that wasn't the job for me. I wanted to be a U.S. Senator. And for that to happen, I had to take on a politically polished and well-heeled opponent: H. John Heinz III, the "Prince of Ketchup."

Powerful people on the Pennsylvania Democratic Committee liked me but, of course, we all knew that taking on John Heinz would be a long shot, at best. Nevertheless, I got the overwhelming endorsement of the Democratic Party, won the primary and ran in the general

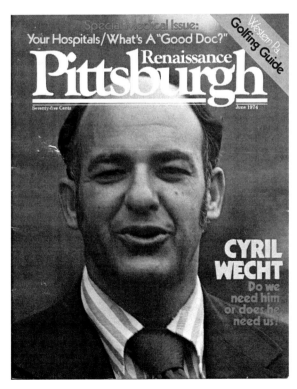

Local luminary, 1974 (*Pittsburgh* magazine).

election against the handsome, young, moderate, incumbent Republican multimillion-aire. That shows you where my head was. But I loved the challenge.

Back in 1982, my interest in politics was keen. And it was in August of that year that Tim Uhrich was forced into the job market after his failed bid to be accepted into law school. His background as a newspaper reporter was a plus, as was the fact that he had worked in the mayor's office of a sizable town. But jobs for people with his skills were hard to come by in those days. One day, however, Tim ran into a friend who told him that she had just been hired to work on a political campaign for a man named Cyril Wecht, who was preparing to challenge John Heinz for his seat in the U.S. Senate. "They're always looking for people at headquarters," she said. "We could use your skills on the campaign. Why don't you come in and talk to us?"

TIM UHRICH: *My first reaction was, "Why would I want to work for a guy who, at least by way of the media, seemed like the biggest asshole on the face of the Earth?" I was reluctant at first, but had to do something to earn at least a meager living. So, finally, on a whim, I went to check things out.*

Our campaign headquarters was located at the University Inn near the Pitt campus, and Tim came by one day and met with a man there named Sal Sirabella, who was running my statewide operation. Sal was a county employee on leave and best known for his political work with Jim and Pete Flaherty, two local political titans, the latter of whom had been Mayor of Pittsburgh.

As it turned out, Sal was planning to get married in October and made it clear to everyone on my staff that he had to leave the campaign in time for his nuptials, in which case someone would be needed to run our operation into the fall. Tim Uhrich figured that, with nothing else to do, and no real employment prospects, he'd get involved with us to see what might happen.

Starting in August, through the end of the election, I spent almost every day with Cyril, helping to run the statewide operation in the day, and traveling with him at night. It was a will-work-for-food type situation. We worked all day and all night for very little, if anything. Cyril was very intimidating at first, because everything in his world seemed, to the uninitiated, to be a bit helter-skelter. It was all very high-intensity and high-impact, just like Cyril.

Tim often says that my speeches in those days were "legendary," so much so that when we would go to events in various counties, which were always a big thing during campaign season, as the Democratic Party's candidate for the U.S. Senate, I was the man everybody wanted to hear.

But everything in 1982 was geared towards Allen Ertel and his race for Governor, and Ertel had a rule: Cyril Wecht could not speak within 20 minutes on either side of him because he feared being overshadowed by Cyril's charisma.

I'll admit that we were often flying by the seats of our pants. And political campaigns can test anyone's nerves, with their tight schedules and almost impossible demands. But I was up for it. I don't really recall this, but Tim remembered one instance in which he and I drove the 50 miles between Pittsburgh and Uniontown in little more than 30 minutes. If true, that might be a record.

TIM UHRICH: *Driving with Cyril always had the potential to be a terrifying experience. When my father, a press photographer in Allentown, came out to visit, he got conscripted into doing some photography work for the campaign. My dad, who was a World War II combat veteran of the Pacific Theater, drove with Cyril and me for one day, after which he told me that he'd never been more afraid in his life. But on some nights, when we were back east, we stayed at my parents' home, and I'll never forget how kind Cyril was to my mother. Thereafter, whenever he would call me, the first thing he would ask is, "How's your mother, Tim?" Or "What are you planning to do for Mother's Day?" Cyril is big on family. No one who knows him would ever question that. Once I had spent some quality time around Cyril, all of my media-fueled preconceptions of him vanished. I found him to be a kind person, and absolutely loyal to a fault.*

Tim's contention is that I have always been loyal to far too many people, many of whom were not worthy of my trust, and this contributed to some of my political problems, not to mention my legal woes. But I've always loved people and have never failed to answer the call when someone needed my help. My friends will attest to that. Consider the night on which I actually brought a dead man back to life.

Once, while out testing the political waters in Southwestern Pennsylvania, I traveled to Lawrence County to speak at a Democratic dinner event that was one of the largest gatherings in the region.

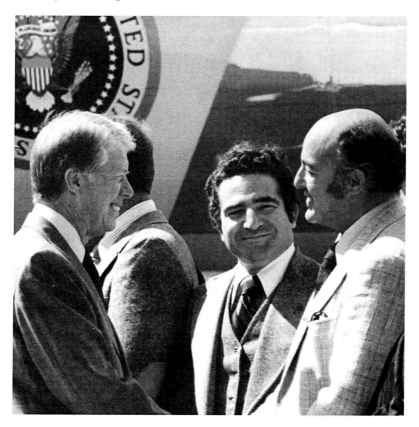

President Jimmy Carter, Beaver County Commissioner Dan Donatella, and me, 1979.

TIM UHRICH: *I wasn't present, but I was told by a colleague that roughly 1,500 people had attended the event at a Masonic hall, or wherever it was. Cyril was giving a speech when a man in the audience had a heart attack and went down. In a flash, Cyril leapt from the dais—he was a doctor after all—performed CPR, and revived the man. The paramedics came, took the guy away, and he survived. And Cyril? He just got back up and continued his speech, picking up where he had left off.*

In the race against John Heinz, I was finally reaching the broad audience I wanted. And as our campaign hurtled toward a close, I was invited to an event in Philadelphia where David Broder, of the *Washington Post*, and a host of other national political correspondents gathered to ask questions of a large scope. I did my best, which was pretty good for a prospective U.S. Senator.

TIM UHRICH: *Cyril did well if he was asked intelligent questions and was allowed to speak his mind. Walter Mondale [Jimmy Carter's Vice President] was quoted in the press once as saying that Cyril was perhaps the greatest political stump speaker in America—and he probably was.*

I only raised about $250,000 for the campaign, which was enough to produce maybe a couple of local television commercials. But I managed to capture 41 percent of the vote, which wasn't too shabby for a balding, middle-aged, Jewish liberal from

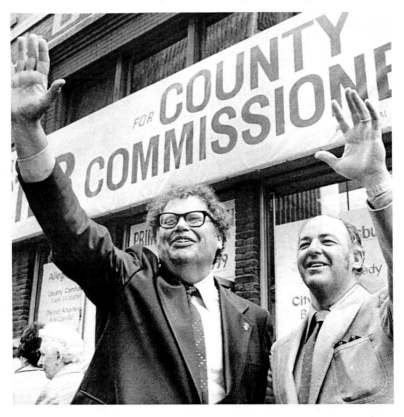

Political triumph, with Allegheny County Commissioner Tom Foerster, 1980 (*Pittsburgh Post-Gazette*).

the Lower Hill District. Not that I thought I had much of a chance against the power and wealth of John Heinz, but had there been a miracle or some freak occurrence, and I had to run against some no-name, replacement Republican candidate, what would have happened? I don't know. But my family and I would have had a very different life. We'd have been fine, I'm sure. "U.S. Senator" was the only political position that I ever really wanted; the only one for which I would have been willing to change my family's lifestyle.

TIM UHRICH: *After the loss in the U.S. Senate race to John Heinz, the knives came out and the powers of the Democratic Party cut Cyril down.*

Sadly, my loss to John Heinz, along with the bad press that had been generated during my first public corruption trial a few years before, led me to lose my County Commissioner's seat in the election of 1983.

TIM UHRICH: *Tom Foerster sensed that Cyril had been damaged and rallied everyone against him. And that was essentially the end of Cyril's political career, beyond the Coroner's Office.*

STUART GRODD: *I never understood why Cyril would have wanted to be a U.S. Senator. He had a marvelous practice. He was writing books. He had four growing kids. He would have had to give up probably $400,000 of income per year for $125,000. Why would he*

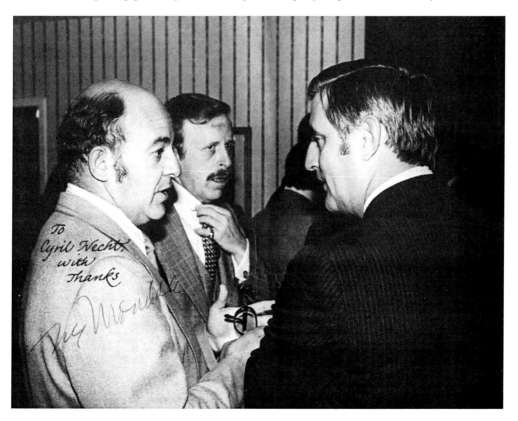

Me, attorney Jack Doherty, and Vice President Walter Mondale, 1984.

ever give that up? What motivated him to want the job? Personal recognition? Love of country? I think he liked the attention. He always liked to be in the public eye. And Cyril's next step would have probably been Vice President of the United States. I don't know if he ever could have made President, being a Jew, but V.P. would have been no trouble. He would have been like Joe Lieberman.

FRANCIS SHINE: *I believe that, if he had become a U.S. Senator, Cyril would have gone to Washington and tore that place apart. Those guys wouldn't have known what to do with him.*

JIM RODDEY: *Cyril would have been a good Senator because he's smart. He would have understood the issues. Couldn't you just see him on the Sunday morning political talk shows? He'd have been on every one, every week, if they would have him.*

SIGRID WECHT: *Losing that race didn't bother me much. I have to admit that I've never enjoyed the political scene, locally or elsewhere. Politicians will kiss you and then stab you in the back.*

After my loss to John Heinz, I vowed (perhaps with two fingers crossed behind my back) that I would no longer be involved in politics. I did, however, and for whatever reason, run unsuccessfully for Pennsylvania State Democratic Chair in 1984 but—until I ran for Coroner again in 1995—and won—I told myself, "That was it." Or so it would have seemed.

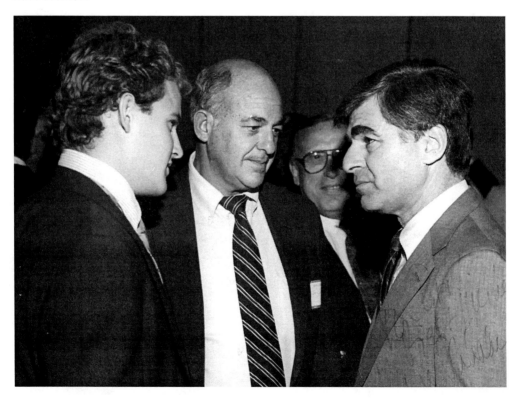

My son, Ben, and me with Massachusetts Governor (and U.S. Presidential candidate) Michael Dukakis, 1988.

In 1999, I decided to run for the newly created position of Allegheny County Executive, and defeated one-term minority County Commissioner Mike Dawida in the Democratic primary. When I ran for the office, as always, I was a Democrat; a social liberal. And it bothered me that some of the Jewish leaders in town, who were also registered Democrats, came out for Jim Roddey, a prominent Republican businessman, who was making his first bid for elective office. But that was par for the course.

JIM RODDEY: *My first knowledge of Cyril was reading about him. I came to town in 1978 and, of course, by then he was a well-established political figure, having been elected Coroner, and then a County Commissioner. For several years, I got involved in a lot of activities in the community. Then I decided to run for office and managed to get the Republican nomination for Allegheny County Executive.*

During the race, Jim and I had the opportunity to learn about each other through a series of 13 debates. I enjoy debating and I'm pretty good at it, going way back to my college days.

JIM RODDEY: *I loved debating Cyril. I enjoyed listening to him because, as everyone knows, he really can talk. He would pontificate on issues, but I learned that he had "hot buttons," and I could hit one of those and set him off on a tirade about something totally unrelated to whatever we were talking about. Through those 13 debates, however, I grew to understand him a bit. There's not a lot of "in between" with Cyril. People either love him or they don't. But in life, you don't accomplish much without making friends and detractors, especially in politics.*

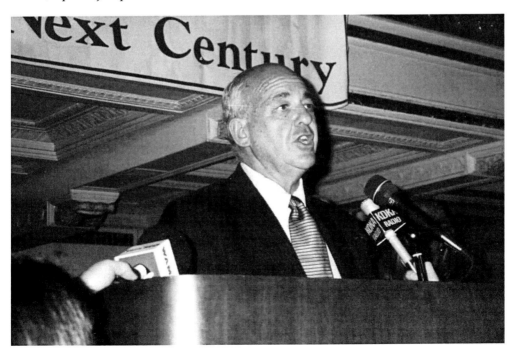

Campaigning for Allegheny County Executive, 1999.

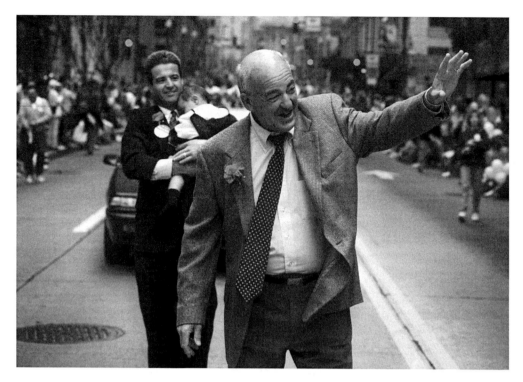

A local favorite campaigning, 1999 (*Pittsburgh Post-Gazette*).

At that point, my life had become a lot about politics, perhaps more than I ever intended, and my involvement did create complications for other pursuits, namely my work in forensic science and running my own consulting business. But look, I was certainly as bright as, or perhaps more, than many of the people who were holding these important public positions. And I believed that a person like me, coming from where I'd come, should have the opportunity to participate.

JIM RODDEY: *Obviously, Cyril is very bright. I don't know what his IQ is, but it must be off the charts. He was good at anything he tried, whether it was playing the violin, practicing medicine, or whatever. He's highly educated and accomplished, but his life was becoming more defined by politics than by anything else. It was a love-hate relationship. On one hand, he loved it, and I can understand that. When you are actually accomplishing things and seeing results from your efforts, it's pretty satisfying. But then there's the purely political side, which is absolutely awful.*

When it came to political debates, I never really prepared in any conventional sense. Maybe I'd jot some notes on an index card or two. But I was well-read and well-informed, and possessed knowledge enough to talk about any issue that was presented, with any opponent. I also had the flair of a performer, and more than enough attitude to go toe-to-toe with any and all comers.

JIM RODDEY: *Cyril never prepared for our debates. He always assumed that he knew more than I did. But as I got to know him, I realized how much he cared about his family, and how much he cared about the community, particularly about people who didn't have the opportunities that many of us have had. I think he's always been proud of the fact that he came from humble beginnings. He was pleased with what he had accomplished. And I don't think he ever has had a great deal of respect for people who inherited their money and rose to a place in life without a lot of effort.*

HOP KENDRICK: *Cyril had always been a very outspoken guy. He was never one to bite his tongue. He cared about people. Nobody could ever attack him on his views about the need for justice or civil rights. He was very concerned about them before many of us were. When he went into politics, particularly when he was Coroner, he won the highest percentage of the African American vote in the history of Allegheny County. No one before or since has ever equaled it.*

WILLIAM ROBINSON: *By far, in terms of a white politician collecting black votes in the county, Cyril was at the top, and it worked to his advantage sometimes. In this county, in the black community, the "Wecht" name is golden. But it has also worked to his disadvantage because some people probably characterized him as a "nigger lover," which may have prevented him from doing some of the things he wanted to do.*

JIM RODDEY: *Cyril could be arrogant and pigheaded, but he had a lot of good qualities, too, and I began to like him. That's difficult to do in a political campaign, particularly when you get attacked about everything you say. In the end, I won the election by a very small margin, and ironically, I won in the 7th and 14th wards, where Cyril lived. In fact,*

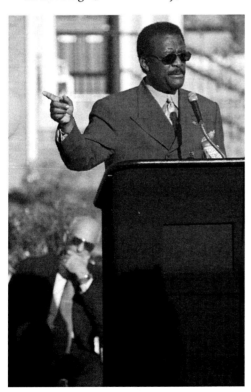

I won in the precinct where he voted. I was very happy to tell Cyril that my margin of victory came from those places. I can also tell you that one of the reasons I beat Cyril was because he invited [O.J. Simpson's chief defense counsel] Johnnie Cochran to Pittsburgh for a campaign event. This is strictly hearsay, so I don't know if it's true or not, but Cyril's handlers didn't want Cochran to come and advised against it. But Cyril wanted it. So, they made a compromise of sorts. "Fine. We'll have him come, but we won't make a big deal of it. We won't put out a press release or promote it much." Well, we found out that Cochran was coming and put out our own press release; "Be sure to see Johnnie Cochran in the Hill District at this time, on this day."

When I was running for Allegheny County Executive, I asked Johnnie Cochran to come in for a fundraiser, which actually turned out to be a foolish and stupid thing to do on my part because it probably cost me the election. I did not realize the depth nor the intensity of the antipathy that

O.J. Simpson's chief defense counsel Johnnie Cochran stumps for me in Pittsburgh, as I look on, 1999 (*Pittsburgh Post-Gazette*).

many white people felt for Johnnie because of the Simpson case. Looking back, it's un-believable to me that I didn't realize that.

TONY NORMAN: *I made fun of the fact that Johnnie Cochran was coming to town in one of my columns, and Cyril was really angry with me. I mocked the idea, not understanding why Johnnie should have anything to say about our local race for County Executive. It seemed to me an overreach on Cyril's part, as if he was saying, "Hey, I know some celebri-ties. Vote for me." In a more generous moment, I figured that Johnnie Cochran might have said, "Good luck with your campaign, Cyril, and if there's anything I can do to help, let me know. I could get the folks in the Hill District excited to turn out." That's probably how it went. I'm sure that Cyril never said to himself, "What I really need to get me over the hump is the endorsement of Johnnie Cochran."*

JIM RODDEY: *Johnnie Cochran arrived in a 20-foot long, white limo and stepped out wearing a lavender suit, and it seemed like every camera in town was there. At that point in the race, all of the rank-and-file union people were probably going to vote for Cyril, but there were a lot of defectors after that. Enough people who were going to vote for Cyril decided to vote for me because of Johnnie Cochran, and that made the difference. The elec-tion could have turned on that one issue.*

WILLIAM ROBINSON: *Bringing Johnnie Cochran in was big miscalculation, and it prob-ably did cost Cyril the election. I think there were people who felt that it was somehow going to work to Cyril's advantage in the black community, and maybe it did. But that's not where Cyril's challenge was. He needed votes in the white community, among people who probably believed that O.J. Simpson was guilty.*

JIM RODDEY: *In our race for County Executive, I got 3 percent of the African American vote. Cyril got 97 percent. He had those votes, without Johnnie Cochran. What I think Cyril admired about Cochran is the fact that, regardless of who he was defending, he did all he could for his clients. I think O.J. was guilty as hell, and I think 99 percent of the American people think that, but Cyril liked the idea that Johnnie had won. He beat the government. He beat the system.*

In all fairness, Jim Roddey ran a pretty good race. But it does pain me a little to think that, had I not misjudged the Johnnie Cochran situation, I may have been elected Allegheny County's first County Executive. But Roddey's team unleashed other forces that hit me pretty hard as well.

JOHN MCINTIRE: *Roddey was smart to have hired political ad man John Brabender, who had done work for Rick Santorum, David Vitter, and a lot of the right-wing nuts that were running around the country in those days. Brabender produced a political ad for Roddey that featured quotes from some of the venomous letters Cyril had written to his enemies over the years: one line here; one line there. I don't even think there was an audio track. It was Cyril's words coming back to haunt him. The ad created the impression that, "This Wecht guy is really angry. I'm not sure if we want him leading the county." I don't agree with that, but it was an effective ad.*

But on the lighter side, Brabender later put together several public service an-nouncements for an educational group, and hired John McIntire to get Roddey and me to zip around Kennywood Park like we were 12-year-old school chums saying some-

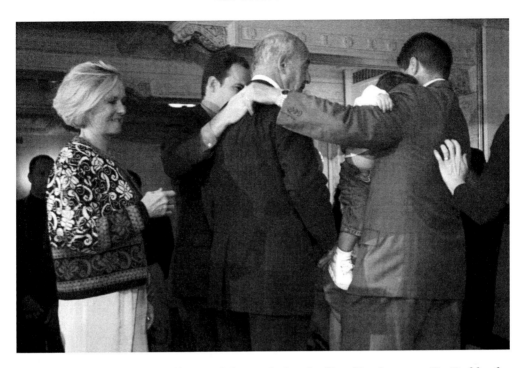

Being consoled by my family after my defeat at the hands of local businessman Jim Roddey for the Allegheny County Executive post, 1999 (*Pittsburgh Post-Gazette*).

thing like, "If we all come together, we can help the educational community." The PSA was cute and I think a lot of people liked it.

> JOHN MCINTIRE: *To his great credit, Cyril did it all with a smile, showing up at Kennywood at 8:00 a.m. on a weekday. I just love that about him. He is an incredible ham, as everybody knows.*

> DAWNA KAUFMANN: *It's very cool to see how well-regarded Cyril is in public. Once, while walking down a Pittsburgh street, a car pulled over, double-parked, and its driver ran over to get Cyril's autograph. In airports, people stop him for photos and to discuss his cases, and Internet message boards devoted to true crime sing his praises and promote his appearances. Dr. Cyril Wecht is "America's Medical Examiner," and there will never be another one like him.*

> JIM RODDEY: *Cyril should be playing more regularly on the national stage. Our stage is too small.*

I didn't miss anything by not becoming County Executive. But believe it or not, I had thoughts about running for Governor of Pennsylvania as late as 2011. I probably would have won the Democratic primary and I think I had a chance to win the whole thing because my name recognition throughout the state was huge. But could I have done that at 80 years old? I'm not sure. And I don't think about it anymore. I probably wouldn't have liked the job anyway.

To this day, I contend that, had I been independently wealthy or perhaps more selfish, I might have dug in politically even more than I did throughout my career. But I

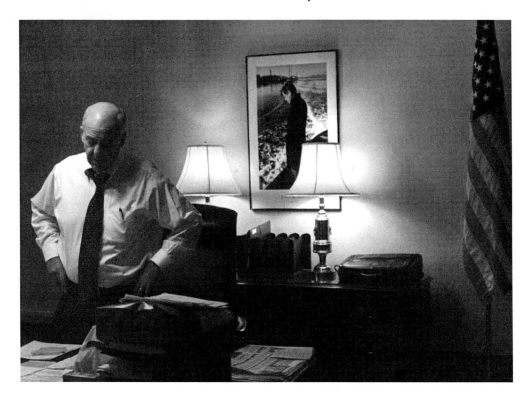

A quiet moment at the end of a long political career, 1999 (*Pittsburgh Post-Gazette*).

was always in the position of having to earn a living. I had four kids in private schools, which cost a lot, so I couldn't throw caution to the wind and go into politics full-time. Even when I was a County Commissioner, I had to do private medical-legal consultations, testify in civil and criminal cases, and do private autopsies to keep the bills paid. I've been doing that from day one and have never stopped. And even when I ran for the U.S. Senate, I had to discharge all the duties of a County Commissioner while, at the same time, keeping up my private practice, and doing some teaching and writing.

Through the years, there were times when I thought about maybe moving to another city and trying my hand at politics elsewhere. But if one is a forensic pathologist by profession, it's not very easy to pick up, move and run for a coroner's position in another community, starting from scratch, as an unknown. I could have gone that route, but would have to have done it many years ago, when I was a much younger man.

Maybe I should have jumped deeper into politics in Pittsburgh or Allegheny County. But, in any case, I've worked hard for a very long time, in and out of the city and county, made a name for myself, and some money. But I never worshipped the dollar or sought to be famous, no matter what anyone says, especially members of the local media. If I had, there are many things I could have done to make more and to be more. And so, here I am.

By way of my reputation and connections, I've had plenty of opportunities. What I will admit without hesitation is that, if you have enough money, you can do certain things in this world and reach people much more easily. For that reason alone, I suppose, like anyone, I would have liked to have been rich. But that's not what makes me tick.

In the United States of America, we adhere to the Golden Rule: "He who has the gold, rules." Look at the U.S. Senate today. I'll bet you that two-thirds of its members or more are multimillionaires. What does that tell you? But had I been born into a wealthy family, I wouldn't be the person I am today. Growing up with less is part of what made me who I am.

Federal Trial Part II

Mad Dogs at the Door

On January 28, 2008, I awoke early to yet another cold, gray winter day in Pittsburgh. It was hard for me to believe that, just a few months shy of my 77th birthday, when many people my age are playing golf in Florida and reminiscing about the high points of their lives, I was at one of my lowest. Powerful forces had aligned against me: from a megalomaniacal local DA to a disgraced FBI agent, not to mention a cadre of bloodthirsty federal prosecutors. My enemies had boxed me in, making it necessary for me to defend myself against a set of ludicrous "criminal" charges. Even if the allegations had been true, the damage to Allegheny County amounted to only a paltry sum of money that I could have easily repaid to get the government off my back. But that's not what they were after.

RICHARD THORNBURGH: *There are two aspects to look at with respect to the case against Cyril Wecht, the first of which was the involvement of Stephen Zappala, of which I know nothing, although I've heard Cyril go on, at some length, about it. Secondly, the record indicates that there was, at that time, an over-intrusion of political considerations in many of the operations at the U.S. Department of Justice. I didn't know about them independently, but I'd read about them in the press. It seemed that U.S. Attorneys were being hired and fired, and cases were going forward or being dropped for partisan political reasons. It was not a healthy environment and I recognized it because I'd worked in the Department of Justice for half of my professional career.*

JERRY MCDEVITT: *Mary Beth Buchanan and Steve Zappala always had some sort of a relationship, largely because of drug cases. If Zappala got a drug case in the state court, especially if it involved crack cocaine, he'd send it down the street to the Feds to prosecute. There's not really much question to me that this all started in Zappala's office. They had conducted the investigations related to the Dixon case and all the rest, then had the case turned over to the Feds rather than prosecuting it themselves.*

I believed that then, and I believe it now. Unfortunately, we were precluded from putting on any evidence to that effect. Zappala wanted to dramatically limit or eliminate the Coroner's power, and I refused to allow it.

MARK RUSH: *Anything that the U.S. Attorney's Office did or did not do rested at the feet of Mary Beth Buchanan. She was the U.S. Attorney, after all. In addition, Steve Stallings, the lead prosecutor for Cyril's trial, struck me as someone who was rabid in his belief in their case.*

Mary Beth Buchanan had been appointed by Arlen Specter, one of Pennsylvania's U.S. Senators in those days. I believe that hers was a purely political appointment because Specter wanted to be remembered for, among other things, appointing the first female U.S. Attorney in Western Pennsylvania history. In any case, Buchanan believed that she needed the scalp of a high-profile Democrat to win points at the Department of Justice, and she hoped that it would lead her to, perhaps, a seat on the Third Circuit Court of Appeals.

RICHARD THORNBURGH: *As far as Ms. Buchanan goes, there's no smoking gun in terms of her motivation for bringing the Wecht case, but there's a strong suspicion that she saw this as a trophy, one that would substantially add to her prestige: bringing down a major public figure.*

None of this was chiseled in stone, but you could kind of put two and two together. That's why I got involved; that and the fact that I had known Cyril for many years, and we'd always been friendly. I never want to see anyone get a bad rap, especially someone I knew well and liked.

Buchanan had a lot riding on what my lawyers and I believed was a bogus case. And while we didn't think we needed luck to beat the charges that had been leveled against me, we were unlucky when it came to the judge assigned to hear my case: the loathsome Arthur J. Schwab.

Arthur Schwab was born in Pittsburgh, attended evangelical Grove City College, and received a Juris Doctor from the University of Virginia School of Law in 1972. He served itinerantly with firms in private practice for 30 years until, on January 23, 2002, pushed by arch-conservative U.S. Senator Rick Santorum, he was nominated by President George W. Bush for a seat on the U.S. District Court for the Western District of Pennsylvania. Schwab was confirmed by the U.S. Senate on September 13, 2002, to the sound of one hand clapping. That hand belonged, again, to the equally loathsome Santorum (who would soon be trounced and evicted from his U.S. Senate office by Pennsylvania voters).

Of all the things I had heard about Arthur Schwab (none of which were good), two things stood out: (1) He was a favorite of Rick Santorum, who had to resort to a near hissy fit in the Senate to get him confirmed; and (2) He had presided over comedian Tommy Chong's trial for an almost laughable "conspiracy" to distribute "drug paraphernalia," sentencing Chong to nine months in federal prison, and adding a hefty financial penalty. I can't say that I knew much about "Cheech and Chong" as a comedy duo, but I did get to speak with Tommy Chong, and I knew this much about his case: He got screwed, royally. The strange thing was that the only U.S. Attorney interested in pursuing charges against Tommy for, essentially, selling pipes for smoking weed, was none other than our very own Mary Beth Buchanan.

After the usual rigmarole and coercion that ensues when people are over-charged under federal statutes, Tommy Chong decided to plead "guilty" which, I'm sure, was what Buchanan hoped he would do. Why did he do it? Because the prosecutors had threatened to go after his family, too, if he didn't. Democrat or Republican, conservative or liberal, this is the way federal prosecutors abuse their power. They're vicious.

JERRY McDEVITT: *Nobody liked Schwab, even when he was in private practice. But now that he was on the bench, he had some power and authority. We reviewed all of his Third Circuit opinions and couldn't believe the number of times he had been reversed for doing exactly the same thing he was trying to do in Cyril's case: issuing rulings without reason or without explanation; and not explaining why he was disregarding Third Circuit law. Schwab had to be the most reversed judge in the history of the Third Circuit. He's notorious for this down there.*

Leading up to my trial, the prosecution tried to squeeze me the same way they did Tommy Chong in an effort to get me to plead "guilty" to at least one charge, and two of my sons, David and Ben, had to hire attorneys. I had paid each of them to work for me, legitimately, but the Feds chose to see it differently. They hoped to accuse me of transferring money to my sons on the bogus theory that they would have paid a lower tax rate on it than I would have. It was all bullshit. But the Feds chose to pressure my sons as part of the net they had cast for me.

State and local prosecutors are not so wonderful either. But they don't have the power of the Feds. They can't dig into your tax history, for example. But when it comes to federal prosecutors, the IRS is used ruthlessly as a weapon and a tool for leverage. Sure, state and local prosecutors might contact the IRS on some major cases to see what dirt they might dig up against defendants or key witnesses, especially expert witnesses, but such requests are few and far between. During the famous O.J. Simpson trial, my colleagues Dr. Michael Baden and Dr. Henry Lee, for the first time in their lives, were audited by the IRS. Those audits were almost surely initiated by the prosecution.

RUGGERO ALDISERT: *I felt that Cyril was being singled-out politically. In my opinion, the charges weren't justified, and I speak about this passionately, as a judge who knows federal law and was involved in the federal courts. Many of Cyril's difficulties stemmed from the fact that he had been Chairman of the Allegheny County Democratic Party. That's part of it. But he is also not a quiet person and sometimes makes statements that antagonize people, which didn't help.*

JERRY McDEVITT: *There was no question that Cyril had done some private work in the County Coroner's Office. For example, lawyers would get a microscopic slide or something for which they needed a determination, so they'd run it up to the Coroner's Office while Cyril was there working, and he'd put the slide under the microscope. Cyril had looked through a county-owned microscope at a slide related to one of his private cases. That was supposedly a "criminal act."*

Ridiculous as this was, in our estimation, it shouldn't have mattered. At the outset, Jerry McDevitt knew that the search warrants issued for the investigation against me were invalid, and presented those facts to Judge Schwab. But Schwab didn't want to find them so. Remember, he had come down the same Santorum-lined path of nomination as Mary Beth Buchanan: the right-wing arm of the Republican Party. The last thing

Schwab was going to do was embarrass the Bush Department of Justice that had just appointed him to the bench. So, he summarily rejected our motion to have the invalid search warrants thrown out, which would have killed my trial before it had even started. As Jerry McDevitt has said, the warrants hadn't been particularized. Investigators must tell you, in writing, what they are searching for. What did the Feds do? They staged a "raid" of my office on a day when we were conducting a coroner's inquest, which always drew the news media. Before the cameras, the Feds seized hundreds of files of old cases in which I had been privately consulted by attorneys from throughout the U.S. They even seized my textbooks.

> JERRY MCDEVITT: *When I saw that the search warrants were invalid, I thought, "Schwab might not be a bad choice for this because he's conservative." Presumably, if you're a conservative judge, you wouldn't like the idea of the authorities barging into someone's office and rooting around for anything they chose. You would uphold the U.S. Constitution. But Schwab couldn't have cared less. He wanted to see Cyril go down, and he tailored everything to try to get a conviction. The thing that was bizarre about Schwab was that you couldn't engage him. You couldn't get him to interact with you. He could have said, "Give me a complete argument telling me why you believe that the search warrants are invalid so I can address it." He never did anything like that. He'd go back and write some stupid opinion and we'd constantly be saying, in reconsideration motions, "Judge, you didn't even address the issue. We're entitled to have you address the arguments that we present to you." Ninety percent of the arguments we presented to Judge Schwab were never addressed. He just denied them. It was a complete "railroad job."*

I was being railroaded all right. Schwab was doing all he could to make it difficult, even impossible, for my defense. It was like an Orwellian nightmare.

> JERRY MCDEVITT: *Before the trial, I think Cyril was worried. When you face 84 counts, all you have to do is get convicted on one. But as a trial goes on, you kind of get a feel for things. You can watch the jury, for example. Anyway, I remember thinking, "What if we don't win? What if Cyril is convicted of something?" But given the legal defense we had raised regarding the invalidity of the charges in the first place, I believed that we'd win ultimately, no matter the verdict.*

Jerry knew that if, down the line, we could get a "real" judge to listen to our argument about the search warrants, there was no way the court would sustain them.

You'll recall that, after three years of shelling out cash to prepare to defend against 84 charges, the prosecution decided to drop 41 of them just two weeks before my trial began. I wasn't unhappy about it, but when I think about how much of my nest egg was spent preparing to fight all 84 charges, it still pisses me off.

> JERRY MCDEVITT: *The rules of the trial were stacked against us. On any given day, after the trial day was over, the prosecution was required to give us a list of their next day's witnesses. There were always 10 or 15, and we knew they weren't going to be able to call that many. They were just screwing with us so we couldn't get prepared. It was so bad that we literally didn't have time to eat. At lunchtime, Schwab gave us just 30 or 40 minutes. We had lunch meat brought in to us and I'd throw a couple of pieces of ham into my mouth, then we'd head back in only to receive the prosecution's witness list at five o'clock. We had to*

prepare until three or four in the morning to cross-examine 10 to 15 witnesses, go home, and then get up and do it all again.

My trial was not an example of how proper trials are conducted. Schwab ran it the way he saw fit and trusted that, with some help from the bench, the government could put me away for a long while.

JERRY MCDEVITT: *In a sidebar once, late in the week, when I was dog-tired, I got into an argument with Schwab. I was sighing because he was doing his usual bullshit when I said to him, "You know what your problem is, Judge? You've never tried a case. If you had ever tried a case, you wouldn't conduct yourself this way." He said, like a kid, "I'll bet that I've been in a courtroom more than you have," to which I responded, "You're doing everything you can to make our lives miserable because we're defending Cyril Wecht." Everything Judge Schwab did was calculated.*

During the trial, one thing that we had to do was challenge the prosecution's nonsense about my use of the county fax machine for the benefit of my private business. I didn't recall doing that very often but, if I did, it was nickel-and-dime nonsense. Incidental faxes are sent every day by government officials. Some operate secondary businesses to supplement their meager public wages. Is doing so criminal? Why couldn't they have just tallied up what they thought I owed the county for faxes and handed me a bill? My attorneys reconstructed from phone records how much I had supposedly "stolen" from the county by sending faxes for my private business. As it turned out, I could have paid off the debt with pocket change.

MARK RUSH: *I totaled up the wire charges for the jury, the "old school way," on yellow paper, just to make sure that they completely understood. The cost of all the actual wires in question came to $3.96. That's all. The government wanted to argue that they were not charging for the cost of the wires, but they were. For what else could they have been charging? For the time it took to send them? Their argument was that Cyril benefited by sending faxes for his outside business which, by the way, isn't illegal. The reaction of the jury to the total cost was telling.*

STANLEY ALBRIGHT (JUROR): *The most important part, as far as I was concerned, was the fact that I could see no crime. If Cyril Wecht spent the county's money on his business, why aren't they just asking him for that money back? Why are they saying he's a criminal? They knew that he had his own business and had told him that they wanted him to be at the Coroner's Office. So, how was it that he was not going to conduct at least some of his private business in that office?*

Mary Beth Buchanan thought the charges that the Feds referred to as the "motherlode" were the private mail fraud charges they had brought against me for supposedly billing people for limousine service to the airport when, in fact, sometimes I didn't take a limo. Each time I traveled for a case, my expenses were paid by the client, limo service included, whether I used it or not. The prosecution zeroed-in on limo expenses because I often had a deputy drive with me to the airport in a county-owned car, after which it was returned to the Coroner's Office. Buchanan believed that, for this, I had no defense, and that no jury would acquit me on such charges.

JERRY McDEVITT: *If Cyril had to work on a case somewhere other than Pittsburgh, he'd drive himself to the airport and his deputy would bring the car back. That would be billed to the client as a limo expense. The client didn't care. They'd pay it because they wanted him.*

MARK RUSH: *I went and met with all the various district attorneys with whom Cyril worked regularly to interview them to be witnesses, and to test the waters to see what they thought of Cyril and his services. There wasn't one who wouldn't testify on Cyril's behalf. And they all said, "We plan to continue hiring him, now and in the future." So, we were going to bring in a parade of state prosecutors to testify against the Feds but, ultimately, we didn't have to do it.*

RICHARD THORNBURGH: *The prosecution couldn't get any lawyers to testify against Cyril. Of those who were allegedly the victims of being "ripped off" with phony expense ledgers, not one of them came forward. That tells you something. Cyril was earning enough in his practice. He didn't need to rip people off for fax or limo charges. It was outrageous.*

STANLEY ALBRIGHT (JUROR): *The prosecutors kept hammering on things that I thought weren't important. They kept trying to get one of Cyril's clients to say something bad about him, but they weren't able to do it. Every one of those witnesses said that they would hire him again in a minute.*

It seemed that the government was saying, when I was breathing in a county building, I was breathing "county air," and could not conduct any private business at the risk of being charged with a federal crime. But district attorneys from other counties often came to meet with me in the Coroner's Office to talk about private cases. Were they engaging in criminal activity, too?

MARK RUSH: *One day, when I had one of Cyril's assistants testifying, I asked, "Did the Pennsylvania State Police visit Cyril in the Allegheny County Coroner's Office?" "Yes." "What about the District Attorney of Westmoreland County, Mr. Peck? Did he visit Cyril at the Allegheny County Coroner's Office?" "Yes, he did." Then I asked, "Did these people come in through the back door? Did they come in at night? Did they hide their faces? Did they all realize that they were conspiring with Dr. Wecht to violate federal law?" The jury got the point. And the other point was that Cyril was always in the County Coroner's Office. He was working for Allegheny County. He was so busy he couldn't leave. The other counties had to come to him.*

Many of the district attorneys' offices in Southwestern Pennsylvania consulted with me, about a half-dozen or so, I guess. I was important to them. After all, I was helping them to solve cases, which was their goal. And all of them decided to continue using me—even during my trial.

Throughout the ordeal, I continued to consult and work on Fridays, when court was not in session, and every weekend. I testified regularly in homicide cases, some of which were taking place in the very same building as my own trial. And I continued to attend professional conferences, including those of the American College of Legal Medicine and the American Academy of Forensic Sciences. In fact, I remember flying to Washington, D.C., on a Tuesday evening after trial to attend the organization's annual event. I had my faithful assistant, Joe Mancuso, waiting for me in a car outside the conference site and, around 11 p.m., after the speeches and activities had ended, I rendezvoused with Joe and he shuttled me back to Pittsburgh so I'd be ready for my trial on Wednesday morning.

JOHN PECK: *I knew, from informal discussions, that we'd all made the decision to continue using Cyril as an expert witness in our cases. We presumed him innocent, and the cases he was doing for us had nothing to do with whatever difficulties he had with the U.S. Attorney's Office. Cyril was being tried over the winter and, one day, there was a severe snowstorm that led to the closing of the federal courthouse [in Pittsburgh] in the middle of the week. Cyril was scheduled to come out on Friday to testify for us in a homicide case. I usually leave my house about 5:45 in the morning and, by then, Cyril was already on the phone to me saying, "They're closing the federal courthouse. Can you rearrange the trial witnesses so I can come out today?" We in Westmoreland County were not closed, and it worked out conveniently, so we did that. Cyril drove out here in a snowstorm and testified.*

Cyril Wecht gives 100 percent of his energy and talent when he participates in a case. He works hard in terms of analyzing the case and coming to definite conclusions. I never felt that he was tempted to give me a conclusion I wanted that may not have been accurate and truthful. That's the rewarding part of having a relationship with him. You can rely on his honesty and integrity.

DAWN CASHMERE (JUROR): *I didn't know anything about Dr. Wecht before the trial; nothing at all. I'm from Seattle, Washington. That's where I grew up, and that's why I had never heard of him. But I came to learn that, through his trial, the man kept working, which clearly showed that people had faith in who he was—and not just his name; they knew him as a person. He never missed a step through the entire trial. That's how Dr. Wecht operates, and it impressed me.*

I had faith that my attorneys would be able to paint a picture to the jury of me as a person and a professional whose very existence was dedicated to forensic science, and discovering the truth. It was clear what I was doing for Allegheny County, and also what I was doing for surrounding counties. DA after DA, state trooper after state trooper; they all came in and spoke about some of the more heinous crimes on which I assisted them. I was confident that many witnesses were going to say, "Without Cyril Wecht, I don't know if we would have gotten convictions."

JERRY MCDEVITT: *By the time we got to trial, only 41 of the original 84 counts remained. On its charges concerning limousine invoices, the prosecution brought in only two witnesses, both of whom loved Cyril. Those witnesses knew exactly what was happening. The government was trying to use them as a vehicle to get a conviction on at least one charge, and the witnesses didn't want anything to do with it. So, they got on the stand and, even knowing that they were supposedly the recipient of a phony invoice for whatever—$100 for a limo—they said that it was no big deal, and that they would hire Cyril again. But this was probably the hardest part of the case to deal with because the limo company from which the invoices were submitted no longer existed. Cyril's secretary was apparently the one who sent the bills out, so the question was, "Did Cyril know that she was doing this?"*

Eileen Young, my secretary, was a key government witness in this regard. And when dealing with her, I think, the prosecution made one of their biggest tactical mistakes in the trial because they kept the poor woman on the witness stand for seven whole days of testimony, which is a lot.

MARK RUSH: *That was the longest cross-examination I'd done in my entire life. I think I had Eileen on cross alone for two-and-a-half days. I was exhausted, but she was an excellent witness. The government had her on the stand for about four days, so she testified for a long, long time. Frankly speaking, I think Eileen Young was the most important witness for Cyril. The prosecution built their case around her and we built our cross-examination around her, too. Eileen was at the center of everything that Cyril did. She kept his daily calendar. She knew exactly what was happening and when. She knew the "life and times of Cyril Wecht," from soup-to-nuts, and was able to convey to the jury a very clear story that Cyril was a robust county servant. Eileen was able to clearly convey to the jury what a day, a week, or a month in the life of Cyril Wecht was like. When she was finished testifying, there was no question that the people of Allegheny County got more than their money's worth from their Coroner, who I think, at the time, was making only about $80,000 a year.*

EILEEN YOUNG: *My husband was a detective for 43 years and he never saw a witness on the stand for seven days. The first day I went up there, I was shaking like a leaf and hyperventilating. I had no idea what it felt like to be in the witness chair. When I started being questioned, [Assistant U.S. Attorney] James Wilson took over, and was merciless. I could barely articulate answers. He said some things that ticked me off and I thought, "Okay, that's it. I'm here and I'm going to tell the truth. You're not going to intimidate me." My attorney was sitting in the courtroom and got a big smile on her face. She could see when I came into my own and got over the fear. It took me about half-an-hour until I was comfortable answering Wilson's questions.*

I was seated on one side of the courtroom and Eileen was seated on the other, and we weren't allowed to speak to each other. She told me later that, from time to time, Jim Wilson would take her back into a little room in the courthouse and threaten her. He'd scream and say to her, "We think you're lying, Ms. Young. You've been granted immunity, but we can still prosecute you for perjury if you keep telling these lies."

EILEEN YOUNG: *Wilson didn't seem to like the truth, but I said, "I intend to tell the truth, whether or not you like it." During the investigation of Dr. Wecht's files, they were able to collect a lot of documents with my name written on them. I told them when they were prepping me for trial that Dr. Wecht had actually made the government's job easier because, when it came to what I did for him, he insisted that it all be documented. Then the prosecutor said, "So, I understand that you did some private work on county time." I said, "Yes, but I was doing county work on my own time."*

I worked from 10 until 8 every day. We had three or four secretaries, and every protocol that they did, which is all county work, had to be proofread by me. During the day, there were so many interruptions that I felt it would be much easier to take the protocols home after work, sit in my easy-chair and proof them. Sometimes I did that until midnight or 1 a.m., if necessary. Then I said to the prosecutor, "If you're saying I did private work on county time, and county time was from 8:30 until 4:30, then I'm guilty. But for me, county time wasn't from 8:30 until 4:30. I worked at home a lot. They got more than their due time from me."

Eileen knew that I wasn't charging private work to the county. I always kept a private office and a private staff and paid for all of it, including office expenses, myself. This was also documented.

JERRY MCDEVITT: *In the end, Eileen broke down. It was strange because, there was one point when they were questioning her about the [dummied] limo invoices and she said, "It was wrong. I'm so sorry." I was thinking, "This is not good." But attorneys have to know when to stop, and the prosecutors didn't. They kept going to the point where it became painful to watch. They were trying to get Eileen to say that Cyril had told her to do this. They had browbeaten her and accused her of all kinds of things that she hadn't done, trying to get her to betray Cyril.*

Because of what the prosecution had done to Eileen, down the road in our closing argument, Jerry pointed out to the jury: "Remember how they treated Eileen Young for seven days on the stand? If they will do that in a courtroom, imagine what they'll do when nobody's watching." Prosecutors hold the power to grant immunity from prosecution, and they did that for Eileen, hoping that she would provide testimony that would help them to convict me. And the judges of whether or not a witness had complied with this responsibility are the prosecutors alone. So, if you don't say exactly what they think you should say, they can claim you didn't testify truthfully, and vacate your immunity. Then they'll often threaten to prosecute you for perjury. The government has a mighty and frightening litigation advantage. When a juror understands how the immunity process works, who would support that? It naturally skews a witness' testimony.

DAWN CASHMERE (JUROR): *I'm a sensitive person and I didn't like the way they attacked Eileen Young. To grill her for seven days was really overkill. I don't know how she made it through.*

◆ ◆ ◆

SISTER GRACE ANN GEIBEL: *I met Dr. Wecht in 2003 when I was still the President of Carlow University. It came up in conversation that he needed a place to do autopsies for his private clients. "I can do them in a garage, Sister. I could do them in Schenley Park under a tree but, if I had a proper place to do my autopsies, then I would really have a base of operation." I was thinking to myself. "Imagine having somebody like Cyril Wecht on the premises. Interested students could learn from him." That's how everything started.*

One day, I was speaking with Sister Grace Ann about what I did for a living and how I did it when, out of curiosity, I asked about a building that Carlow had opened in 1998. She invited me to come and take a tour. Afterwards, I told her, "It's state-of-the-art. Pitt doesn't have anything like it."

SISTER GRACE ANN GEIBEL: *The building is referred to as "Science and Technology." We put all the science labs in it, and as much of the technology as possible related to our computer science program. One day, I said to Cyril, "I don't see why you couldn't use the building for your autopsies, but I'll need to check how much it's being used and how much the faculty needs it."*

Carlow University had a connection with Shadyside Hospital for respiratory therapy. As I recall, that was about the only thing for which the building was being used. They kept a cadaver there and would open the place up for science majors to do dissections, or what have you. The building seemed ideal to me for my purposes, and Sister Grace Ann agreed.

SISTER GRACE ANN GEIBEL: *Cyril said he just needed a place to do autopsies, and could do about 300 a year. "We could really build a course of study around that," I thought. So, we talked on the phone forever. It took about three or four years to get the curriculum the way he wanted it. That's one of the things I learned about how Cyril functions. He's a perfectionist to the "nth" degree, and never leaves a stone unturned. For Carlow, it was a great opportunity, as it was for Cyril. And all the while we were working on this, Cyril never once mentioned money. Anybody who hears this will think I was the most irresponsible administrator ever born, but I didn't want to bring up money because I didn't want to put it on a business level, at least at that stage. But I did think, "If Cyril starts asking for the pay that he deserves, we're going to have to discontinue this."*

Designing the curriculum was my job, and Sister Grace Ann lined up the faculty. In any college or university, the faculty have the power to say "yes" or "no" before any significant or substantial new program is launched. You can't really shove anything down the throats of tenured academicians or university administrators and, while I wanted very much for them to say "yes" to my program, I also wanted them to support and promote it while we were getting it up and running.

SISTER GRACE ANN GEIBEL: *Our students were so impressed. I remember once going into an assembly to talk about something or other, when one student asked, "Do you mean that Cyril Wecht is going to be part of the program?" I said, "Yes, you will have access to him." Then she said, "Oh, my gosh!" I said, "Here's what you should do: Get into his course and make sure that he is able to observe what you do. Interact with him as much as possible, then make reference to it on your résumé." I was thinking that, if students could include Dr. Wecht's name on their résumés in a significant way, it would take them places. The students were almost star-struck. I said, "Cyril, they are in disbelief that they're going to have access to you." And he was just as interested in them, and got more and more interested. I could tell that this was the "real deal."*

Universities want to be able to offer as many exciting courses as possible, and having a world-renowned authority teaching one of them was a good draw. I would go to Carlow when parents were in for "Admissions Day," and talk to them. It was no problem because I lived not far away.

SISTER GRACE ANN GEIBEL: *What built up the program was student contact with Cyril. He was a magnet. Students were learning so much and they would tell me so. When we met, I would talk to them, off-the-record, about the program. "Is it really that good? What do you think?" They'd say, "He just knows so much." That's how I knew we had a good thing going.*

During my trial, the prosecution focused on the usual when it came to my interactions with Carlow University: "What was Dr. Wecht getting out of this arrangement?" I'll tell you this: I never got a penny. Sister Grace Ann said so, emphatically, and they were in disbelief. She kept saying that the pay-off for students was going to be astronomical because they were going to be eminently employable. After all, the nation needs well-trained technicians in autopsy work. And there wasn't another program in the country that could have come close to what we had created.

JOE MANCUSO: *Cyril was on the faculty and got to use the space. That was the payback. Unfortunately, the trial nipped things in the bud, because the program was not publicized or advertised after the indictment came down. Other programs were, but the autopsy program wasn't. If it had been, we'd have had 40 or 50 students in every class. It was a great program.*

SISTER GRACE ANN GEIBEL: *When Cyril was indicted, I said to him, "This is an impossibility. They can't be trying you." I kept thinking to myself, "He's not put together that way. Even if he was stupid, he wouldn't have done what they said he did." Then, in the throes of the trial, Cyril asked, "Sister, I don't want to take advantage of us knowing each other, but would you be willing to write a letter for me, sort of like a character reference?" I did and, in that letter, I focused on the fact that Cyril was doing this program with us because that's what he knew and that's what he wanted to give. He has the "flaw of generosity." Cyril is truly the most honest and generous person I think I have ever known. Right after I wrote that letter, I called him up and he became very emotional. He said, "Nobody has said things like this about me since my father." I said, "Cyril, nobody can touch you because you are not guilty. You just have to ride it through." He didn't need me to tell him that. Cyril's a walking example of "the truth."*

Sister Grace Ann was on the stand for about seven hours between one day and the next. She told me that when she looked out at the faces of the FBI agents sitting in the courtroom, all in a block, with their buttoned-up collars and dark suits, she thought, "They're like a pack of mad dogs."

SISTER GRACE ANN GEIBEL: *I was terrorized because I knew how much I did not know when it came to legal jargon and the prevailing lexicon of language. I knew that what I was going to say could be easily discounted and I would probably look like a jerk. At best, I thought I was going to look like an inept administrator. Then I thought, "Who cares?" Mind you, I was never into details; I just liked people. The prosecutors proceeded to place items before me, like a purchase order for two vials of something or other, and then asked, "Have you seen this before?" I would say, "I might have." "Is that your signature there?" "Sure, looks like it." I had no memory of this stuff. You wouldn't remember such details if you were president of a university and thinking of other things such as, "Where is this place going to be in 20 years?"*

At one point, Sister Grace Ann was asked if Carlow University had made an arrangement with me to supply cadavers from the Allegheny County Coroner's Office in exchange for free autopsy space, to which she replied, "I find that question reprehensible." Sister Grace Ann was also asked, "What's your opinion of Dr. Wecht?" This gave her the opportunity to say, kindly, "I hold him in the highest regard." From the looks on their faces, the "mad dogs" were not pleased. But I could see that the jury was with her. Then Jerry McDevitt asked the jury, "Who are you going to believe? A 'woman of God,' or the federal government?"

SISTER GRACE ANN GEIBEL: *Jerry was so helpful because, when I was fumbling around from nerves, he would rephrase my responses and say, "Is this what you meant?" I'd say, "Yes." I was terrorized because I wanted it to go the way it needed to go. I didn't want to do any damage. After my first day on the stand, a woman who lived in the apartment across the hall from me asked, "How did it go, Sister?" I said, "They're mad dogs down there. They're out to get him."*

DAWN CASHMERE (JUROR): *Sister Grace Ann couldn't have described the prosecution better. My main focus was on [FBI agent] Brad Orsini. He kept turning around in his chair and glaring. He was clearly trying to intimidate us and, right away, that turned me off. After a while, I got the impression that they were all snakes. One of the witnesses spoke about how the FBI came to her home to question her on Palm Sunday. That showed me their character. If they couldn't leave someone alone with their family on a Sunday, I couldn't have any respect for them.*

JOHN PECK: *When half the people in Western Pennsylvania are Catholic, the last thing you want to do is question the truth of a nun. As a lawyer, you have to think about that in advance. Every witness is unique and people in positions of moral authority, like clergy, must be treated with respect. All of us who went to Catholic schools knew nuns. Maybe we didn't like them at the time, but they were right and we were wrong more often than not. What a powerful witness Sister Grace Ann was. First, she was religious, and there likely was one or more Catholics on the jury. Secondly, she was a woman, speaking to women on the jury. The prosecution should have dropped the Carlow part of the indictment from the beginning.*

DAWN CASHMERE (JUROR): *I felt bad that they called this older woman out. She was a nun and nuns convey a certain kind of Godliness. The way they questioned her was upsetting to me.*

STANLEY ALBRIGHT (JUROR): *I think Sister was definitely hurt because they were almost calling her a criminal, accusing her of doing something shady, like making some kind of unholy deal with Cyril about cadavers for office space. I saw she had tears in her eyes. I was sitting that close.*

The body-snatching issue was seized upon by the media and was the subject of some of the most horrible cartoons ever. What made them especially horrible was the fact that I believe anti–Semitism was at their core. They made me look wicked and shadowy, like a "Shylock" who was willing to stoop as low as selling human corpses for a handful of shekels. It was sickening.

DAWN CASHMERE (JUROR): *I went into the trial not having feelings either way, so I really had to pay attention to all the evidence, and listen to what everyone had to say. It wasn't until I met with the other jurors to begin deliberating that I would go home and think about it.*

JERRY MCDEVITT: *Judge Schwab would come out to the bench sometimes and say, "I consulted with other judges on this," suggesting that what he was about to do was supported by others. I thought, "If other judges are making the decisions, then let me argue to them." I didn't even know who these judges were, and didn't know what Schwab was telling them or whether he was accurately portraying our arguments. The way he conducted things was just so irregular.*

At one point, juror Stanley Albright, who appeared to be on our side (and I think Schwab and the prosecution knew it), fell ill. He had chest pains and was dispatched to a local hospital for tests. Once the test results were reviewed, his cardiologist cleared him to return, but by then he had been replaced by an alternate juror. This was very odd because earlier, a female juror, who we came to know later was not on my side, was sick for several days, and Schwab waited for her.

STANLEY ALBRIGHT (JUROR): *One of the lady jurors got very ill so they canceled things for a couple of days until she was able to come back. After I got ill, a statement was issued—I don't know by whom—that said I was not able to come back because of the pressure of the trial. I never said anything like that. I don't know who made that up.*

DAWN CASHMERE (JUROR): *They wanted to replace Stanley with someone who would be on their side.*

When the prosecution finished presenting its ludicrously weak case against me, my attorneys and I believed that the government had not met its burden of proof, so it wasn't necessary for us to present any witnesses of our own, and we didn't. The case went to the jury and, as it was explained to me, the first jury vote was 11–1 for "not guilty," which didn't surprise me.

DAWN CASHMERE (JUROR): *From the start, one female juror was determined to vote "guilty."*

STANLEY ALBRIGHT (JUROR): *Everybody was angry at her for holding out. We kept going round and round and, somehow, she managed to get some of the other jurors to side with her. She kept hitting on this: "He was stealing from his employer." To me, if you take too many paperclips home, then you owe your employer some money. But the charge was worded in such a way as to insinuate that Dr. Wecht had committed a crime, and many of us were having a problem with that. That's when she started in: "If you work for somebody and take stuff from the office for your own use, that's stealing; that's criminal." She believed that using the county's fax machine for personal business was criminal, too, so she held out. Before, the vote was lopsided in favor of acquittal, and I was so surprised when I learned that it had changed to about 50/50.*

DAWN CASHMERE (JUROR): *All through the trial, I remained neutral because I hadn't heard all of the evidence or all of the testimony. But when it came time to vote, I laid out my hand: "Not guilty." Five of us had the same thoughts. We were more educated than some of the others, and I think that's what pulled us together. At that point, there were five votes for "not guilty" and seven for "guilty." After that, we weren't getting anywhere. No one was budging. We weren't going to get seven people to come to our side, and we were not going to agree on a "guilty" verdict.*

Juror Dawn Cashmere told me later that, on the day the jury was going to read its verdict, she had a hard time looking at my wife, because she was afraid that Sigrid would look back at her.

DAWN CASHMERE (JUROR): *Mrs. Wecht was looking at us trying desperately to get a feel for which way this thing was going. So, I looked right at her and tried to show her, to tell her, in my own way, that everything was going to be OK. The trial had been grueling for us, and I can only imagine how it was for Dr. and Mrs. Wecht. The court would drag them in whenever we had questions. They'd call Dr. Wecht and he had to drop whatever he was doing and come to court. I have no idea how he survived. Any normal person would have had a nervous breakdown. He had to be so strong to make it through that, and to get his life on track again.*

STANLEY ALBRIGHT (JUROR): *The prosecution built a house with a faulty foundation. They certainly didn't build the case on bedrock; they built it on sand, and it collapsed.*

In the end, a mistrial was declared. The trial was over.

MARK RUSH: *At her news conference after the mistrial, Mary Beth Buchanan basically said that Cyril was guilty but the jury did not convict him. So, we filed a complaint against her with the Office of Professional Responsibility and the U.S. Department of Justice for those comments.*

Buchanan rattled her saber and said she intended to retry me, but that was unlikely to happen, in the estimation of my lawyers. They didn't believe that the U.S. Attorney's Office (or the Third Circuit, for that matter) could handle a second swing-and-miss at me. The first cut was embarrassing enough. What do they say? "Hope springs eternal?" Yes. Even in the courtroom.

To Sin by Silence
The Assassinations of JFK and RFK

June 5, 1968. All was quiet at the Wecht home in Squirrel Hill. My sons—David, Daniel and Ben—and I had all turned in early. Sigrid was resting at West Penn Hospital, having just given birth to our youngest child and only daughter, Ingrid. In the morning, I was set to take the boys to attend a pair of my speaking engagements: one in Washington, D.C.; the other in Puerto Rico. We had planned to be away for several days to allow Sigrid and the baby to return home and get settled free from the usual family commotion. The plan was perfect—until the phone rang at 4 a.m.

On the line was my friend, Dr. Thomas Noguchi, who was, at the time, Chief Forensic Pathologist for the Chief Medical Examiner/Coroner of Los Angeles County. Tom was calling from his office on the West Coast bearing some tragic news. Senator Robert F. Kennedy of New York, who had been on the campaign trail seeking the Democratic nomination for President of the United States, had just been shot, and the situation didn't look good.

> TOM NOGUCHI: *I was awakened just after midnight, turned on the television, and learned that Senator Kennedy had been shot. I knew that, should death occur, I would be responsible for conducting a thorough examination, including an autopsy. So, I called Cyril for advice.*

I was one of the first persons Tom thought to contact once he had received the terrible news about Bobby Kennedy. For Tom, barely into his 40s at the time, the case was sure to be monstrous—much bigger than even the one involving Marilyn Monroe, over which he had presided in 1962. He knew that he had to proceed with caution.

Twenty-five hours later, Robert F. Kennedy died at Good Samaritan Hospital in Los Angeles. So, it proved wise that Tom had elected to get a head start on preparations for the political tumult and media onslaught that would no doubt follow. Tom didn't need advice when it came to the autopsy. But he was well aware of my familiarity with the John F. Kennedy assassination case, and the many mistakes—unintentional and otherwise—that were made handling it. He wanted to avoid a repeat.

> TOM NOGUCHI: *We installed a direct phone line from my office to the hospital so that we could get immediate updates on the Senator's condition. His brain waves went flat around*

8:30 p.m., so I had to make a decision. On Cyril's advice, at midnight, before death finally came at 1:44 a.m., I called for assistance. And we were prepared to do the autopsy that morning.

My main concern was that agents of the federal government would try to pull some of the same stunts with Bobby that they did with John Kennedy, the most critical of which would have been moving the late Senator's body from the Los Angeles County Medical Examiner's Office prematurely, *and illegally*, given that Los Angeles County had jurisdiction in the case. Tom retained me as an official consultant on the Bobby Kennedy matter. Right off the bat, I recommended that he speak with Pierre Salinger, a native Californian who was close to the Kennedy family, and that he stay one step ahead of the Feds by inviting three forensic pathologists, all of whom we knew, from the Armed Forces Institute of Pathology, to witness the autopsy.

Tom Noguchi: *Cyril is a very close friend. Sometimes I feel like he's my brother. I trust and respect him so, if I have a problem, I often call him for advice.*

The assassination of Robert F. Kennedy propelled me into the rarefied air of the media. Before long, journalists began calling on me to take advantage of my expertise: everyone from Dan Rather at CBS News, to local newspaper reporters and newscasters. That's how it's done in America. So began my media career.

My relationship with Tom Noguchi stretched back a number of years and was unique in one eerie respect. On Friday, November 22, 1963, I happened to be in Los Angeles for a private consultation, and was meeting with Tom at the L.A. County Medical Examiner's Office. We were in the autopsy room talking about cases, and thinking about where to go for lunch. All of a sudden, Tom's secretary rushed in, whispered something in his ear, and his face went blank. "The President has been shot," he said with a look of horror and bewilderment. So, we left the office hurriedly and headed to a nearby restaurant that had a television so that we could follow the news. How strange it was that, less than five years later, I would hear the news about the murder of the President's younger brother from Tom as well. Those two horrible and historic cases bonded us.

My involvement in the saga of JFK actually began in the fall of 1964 when, as a recently minted doctor and lawyer, I held the post of Assistant DA and Medical Advisor in the Allegheny County District Attorney's office. The director of the County Crime Lab, which was an integral part of that office at the time, was Charles McInerney, and he and I became friends.

As a young pathologist, I spent most of my time with Charlie dealing with the forensic science aspects of the Crime Lab, which had been established only a few years before. One day, Charlie, who was a Program Co-Chair for the upcoming annual meeting of the American Academy of Forensic Sciences (AAFS), of which I had been a member since 1962, told me that the Academy was planning to conduct a full-day plenary session concerning the Warren Commission and its 888-page final report on the assassination of President Kennedy. That report had been presented to President Lyndon B. Johnson on September 24, 1964, and was made public three days later. It concluded, among other things, that Lee Harvey Oswald acted alone in the killing of John Kennedy and the wounding of Texas Governor John Connally, who was riding in the same car as the President in the Dallas motorcade.

Charlie McInerney explained that the Warren Commission Report would be analyzed at the 1965 AAFS meeting from the perspectives of pathology, toxicology, psychiatry, criminalistics, anthropology, and so on. He then asked a fateful question, one that would change my life and alter the trajectory of my career: "Would you, Cyril, be willing to address the John F. Kennedy assassination case from the pathology angle?" I said, "Yes."

So, in the fall of 1964, I went to the Carnegie Library in Pittsburgh to review the Warren Commission Report, which comprised 26 volumes. To my astonishment, I found that, other than a small and incomplete one at the tail end of Volume 15, it had no index. My contention has always been that the Feds had done this deliberately so that neither the American public nor the news media would bother to read let alone research the report. But no matter. Eventually, I was able to pull together the information that I needed, prepare my presentation and deliver it at the annual conference of the AAFS, in February 1965. And I've been up to my eyeballs with the JFK assassination ever since.

It was the dead of winter in Chicago and, not unexpectedly, the weather was extremely cold. Consequently, nobody from the AAFS meeting was interested in venturing outside the comfortable Drake Hotel for any reason whatsoever. This left me and my fellow presenters with a captive audience. And when I gave my talk, which included my views on the JFK autopsy and the supplemental brain report (the x-rays and photos were under seal at the time), all hell broke loose. There were FBI agents in the audience who were sent there, no doubt, by J. Edgar Hoover, and they did not like my take on the case at all. I made various criticisms of their agency, and others. But this was early on in my investigation, so I barely broached the absurdity of the "single-bullet theory." All I had to go on were the broad strokes of the Warren Commission Report, which provided ample reason to begin poking holes in the government's fairy tale.

That presentation before the membership of the American Academy of Forensic Sciences led to a call from Mark Lane, who wrote the book *Rush to Judgment* about the case. Mark believed, as did I, that it was far from "open-and-shut."

MARK LANE: *The goal of the Warren Commission was to reassure the American people. But the only thing that would have made us happy is if the President had not been killed or, at least, if we gained a degree of certainty that a group of assassins was not still on the loose in America. How did they reassure us? They tried to convince us that it wasn't true. The goal of the Warren Commission should have been to learn the truth. But it was never looking for the truth. They failed in reassuring us because we didn't believe them. And it changed the way Americans would look at announcements by the government from then on.*

Another fellow wanderer along the trail of the truth about the JFK assassination was Josiah Thompson (we call him "Tink"), the author of a fine book about the Kennedy case called *Six Seconds in Dallas*, for which I wrote a special chapter. Tink was instrumental in the expansion of my investigation, because he helped me to secure permission to study, frame-by-frame, the famous Zapruder film at the New York headquarters of Time-Life, where it was being kept. Abraham Zapruder, a private U.S. citizen, became unwittingly and inextricably linked to the JFK assassination by filming, with an 8mm home-movie camera, President Kennedy's motorcade as it passed through Dealey Plaza in Dallas, Texas, on November 22, 1963. As fate would have it, Mr. Zapruder unexpectedly captured the President's assassination on film.

> JOSIAH THOMPSON: *I met Cyril for the first time in 1966. I had been hired as a consultant for* Life *magazine to research the Kennedy assassination. At that point in time, Cyril had taken a position on the case, and was known. So, I worked through the editors at* Life *to get approval for Cyril, myself, and a few other interested parties, to screen the Zapruder film privately. At the time, the only other way anyone could have seen that film would have been to call up the National Archives and travel to Washington, D.C. Then Marion Johnson would screen a dim FBI copy of a Secret Service copy of the film, and it may even have been a copy of a copy, which wasn't worth much [to researchers].* Life *had the original, having purchased it [on November 23, 1963]. The reason I went to work at* Life *was to get access to a really good copy of the Zapruder film, and then to use it to measure movements, and things of that sort.*

Other contacts were made during that time as well, including one with a woman named Sylvia Meagher, the eventual author of another book on the JFK case called *Accessories After the Fact*. Between 1964 and 1965, Mrs. Meagher took on the herculean task of assembling a more comprehensive index for the Warren Commission Report. Bear in mind, this was before computers and word processing. I visited her in New York City and we became good friends. Sylvia had no money to hire assistants, so she did it all by herself. Like me, she knew that something was just not right.

As everyone knows, the Warren Commission concluded that one single bullet produced seven wounds in two men. The bullet supposedly entered President Kennedy's back about 5.5 inches below the crest of his right shoulder, slightly to the right of the midline. According to the Warren Commission, the shot was fired from the sixth-floor window on the southeast corner of the Texas School Book Depository Building by Lee Harvey Oswald. That means that the bullet was traveling from back to front, right to left, and downward. So, we have a bullet striking the President in the back traveling downward from a sixth-floor window and yet, it emerges in the front of his neck 11.5 degrees *above* the level of the entrance wound. To this, some of my colleagues have said, "But what if President Kennedy was bending over?" Of course, that's bullshit because, thanks to Mr. Zapruder and his camera, we know that the President wasn't doing that. We can see clearly where everyone—President and Jackie Kennedy, and Texas Governor John Connally and his wife—was positioned in the car.

The Warren Commission would have had us believe that, next, that same bullet emerged from President Kennedy, veered to the left, then reversed itself in mid-air, and struck Governor Connally in the back, behind his right armpit. Then it traveled through Connally's chest, piercing his right lung and shattering his right fifth rib interiorly, and exited the Governor's chest below the level of the nipple.

According to the single-bullet theory, as presented to the Warren Commission by Arlen Specter (who would later serve as a U.S. Senator from Pennsylvania), that bullet entered Connally from the back in the right side of his rib cage. Based on calculations derived from the Zapruder film, the Governor was struck by a bullet that was traveling 2,100-feet-per-second in initial velocity and slowed down by perhaps a few hundred-feet-per-second at most after traveling through President Kennedy. It then emerged, moving downward 27 degrees, below the level of the nipple, hooked up and around to where John Connally was holding his white Stetson hat, and hit him in the back of the wrist. Finally, the bullet emerged from the front of the Governor's wrist, moved at a downward angle of 45 degrees, and pierced his left thigh. That's the single-bullet theory, folks, a scenario so ridiculous that it was hilariously parodied decades later on the NBC television sitcom *Seinfeld*, and in many other programs.

One thing that makes Arlen Specter's theory so totally absurd is that the bullet in question destroyed four inches of the right fifth rib of John Connally and produced a fragmented fracture of his radius, one of two large bones that connect the elbow to the wrist. Keep in mind, Governor Connally was six-feet-four-inches tall; a big-boned Texan. And despite breaking those two bones in such an extensive fashion, the bullet was discovered in near pristine condition at the end of its fanciful journey. Its only deformity was at its base, and that resulted from the impact of the gun's firing mechanism. The entire copper-jacketed shell was intact. There was no indentation on its nose or its cone. And that, my friends, is highly improbable.

Another key point that blows a gaping hole in the single-bullet theory is the weight of the bullet. In store-bought condition, the bullet in question—a 6.5 mm, copper-jacketed, lead-core piece of military ammunition—was an inch-and-a-quarter in length and one-quarter-inch in diameter with a weight of 161 grains. When it was found, it weighed 158.6 grains, missing only 2.4 grains after traveling magically through two grown men. Two-point-four grains is 1.5 percent of 161. We see fragments in the x-rays of Connally's chest, wrist, and thigh, and possibly in Kennedy's chest, too—little bits, minimally small, but visible nonetheless—yet we are told that all these fragments together constituted only 1.5 percent of the original weight of the bullet.

MARK LANE: *One day, I held a press conference in Washington, D.C. [about the JFK assassination] and the first person I called to be there was Cyril. He sat next to me and, together, we fielded questions, which was great because I'm not a doctor; I'm a lawyer. Cyril was a forensic pathologist, and a good one, so he was just the guy I needed to talk about the Kennedy autopsy report and certain photographic evidence. I remembered Cyril discussing the single-bullet theory on CBS-TV [June 26, 1967]. He was interviewed by Dan Rather and this is what he said, essentially: "In medicine, we never like to say that something is impossible, but it's highly improbable that the Warren Commission was correct about what that bullet did." Cyril totally knocked out the single-bullet theory. As a scientist, he would not say that it was impossible, but he made it clear that he thought it was.*

Let's travel back to November 22, 1963, and review some other key facts that might surprise you regarding the situation surrounding the assassination of President John F. Kennedy. In the immediate aftermath of the assassination, President Kennedy, mortally wounded, was taken to Parkland Hospital in Dallas with no chance for survival. By evening, Trauma Room 1 was lined with FBI and Secret Service agents, and local authorities, ostensibly to supervise the goings-on. In essence, the reaction to the President's death was nothing short of a controlled law-enforcement operation. But why?

Another open question is, "Who made the decision to move the President's body from Dallas?" The Dallas Medical Examiner, Dr. Earl Rose, a board-certified forensic pathologist, was already on site, and he insisted that the autopsy of the President should take place at Parkland, according to the laws of Dallas and the State of Texas, before the body could be released. Nonetheless, the American military essentially confiscated the President's body, in violation of local and state laws, and took it, first, to Washington, D.C., only to decide (they say to honor the wishes of Jackie Kennedy) to conduct the President's autopsy at Bethesda Naval Hospital in Maryland, because John Kennedy had been a Naval officer during World War II. But who *really* made that decision?

In addition, it is still unclear who was responsible for the selection of two Navy pathologists, Dr. James J. Humes and Dr. J. Thornton Boswell, neither of whom had ever conducted a gunshot-wound autopsy, to do the post-mortem examination of our President. It's true that shortly thereafter, as an afterthought, another pathologist was summoned to assist, a physician named Dr. Pierre Finck, whom I knew; an Army man. But, to that date, Pierre's work had been limited largely to reviewing military-related cases in Vietnam, for which few autopsies, if any, were ever performed. He had very little hands-on experience and, like Humes and Boswell, was a poor choice for such an important job.

ROBERT TANENBAUM: *The law required the body to be autopsied in Dallas, and there was a confrontation at the hospital [about moving it]. Why? Dr. Charles A. Crenshaw, a trauma expert who was one of several physicians who assessed President Kennedy's gunshot wounds early on, with some assistants, noted a gaping hole in the back of the President's head, circled it [in a photo] and had people sign off on it. One would be hard-pressed to make something like that up when simply providing observations. Eventually, we [supposedly] saw those photographs, which weren't available for a couple of years, and in them we don't see that gaping hole.*

Dr. Crenshaw also noted that there were entry wounds in the President's neck and throat, and one to the right-front-center of his head. The Warren Commission, of course, did not think it was important to call Dr. Crenshaw as a witness, which bothers the hell out of me. By the way, Dr. Crenshaw and his team were threatened by the director [of the hospital] the next day who said [in essence], "If anybody talks about any of this, their careers will be ruined." That was within a couple of days of the assassination.

For the life of me, I can't understand why anyone would disregard the findings of the Crenshaw group. Now, that wasn't everybody. They did bring in [medical people from the Parkland area] who said, "a tracheotomy was done on President Kennedy, so we couldn't see where the wound was [on his throat]." That's fine. But if you conduct an honest investigation, you have to put that into the record. And you must have [the attending medical people] testify as to what their reasons were for doing what they did.

In a nutshell, this is my theory about what happened to President John F. Kennedy on that sunny, autumn afternoon in Dallas. I believe that an act so precise and profound could not have been the work of a lone gunman. The assassination of our President was a *coup d'état*, and the only people who could have pulled it off were either active or former U.S. military or CIA personnel. It could only have been orchestrated by a host of very secretive people and, a deathbed confession notwithstanding, the truth about who actually pulled the trigger (or triggers) will likely never be known.

> MARK LANE: *We know the truth. The CIA killed President Kennedy. This was not a back-alley killing. This was in Dallas, Texas, on a bright, sunny day. He's got the Secret Service surrounding him, the best protective organization in the world. But let's look at what the Secret Service did. There was [an agent] driving the car. What's his job, if he hears a sound like a "firecracker?" Speed up. Get out of there. What did he do? He slowed down. In the passenger seat to his right was another agent. What was his job? At the first sign of any problem, he was to leap over any obstacles and cover the President's body with his own. All of the Secret Service agents present were assigned to protect President Kennedy, except for Clint Hill. He was assigned to protect Mrs. Kennedy, and probably didn't "get the memo" that day because he wasn't part of the White House detail related to the President. His job was to protect Jackie. He jumped off his car, jogged after the Presidential limousine and caught it. Jackie was trying to escape from the limo and Clint pushed her back in.*

For me, when it comes to the assassination of John F. Kennedy, the arrow on the dial of guilt keeps pointing to the CIA, for a host of reasons. The CIA was at loggerheads with Kennedy about his approach to handling Fidel Castro and Cuba, which the agency saw as appeasement or being "soft on communism." The CIA also resented the President's refusal to provide cover for the Cuban exiles brigade, which had been trained and funded by the U.S. government and the CIA for the invasion of Cuba at the Bay of Pigs in 1961. After that failed attempt to overthrow Castro's regime, the USSR began placing nuclear missiles in Cuba to deter any future attacks by the Americans. The deal made in secret between Kennedy and Khrushchev, which precluded any further attempts to overthrow Cuba, dashed the hopes of both the CIA and the anti–Castro Cuban exile movement. To make matters worse, Kennedy fired CIA Director Allen Dulles and slashed the CIA's budget in 1962, perhaps in retaliation for his belief that he had been lied to time and time again by the agency in an effort to manipulate him into ordering an all-out U.S. invasion of Cuba.

I remember reading that John Kennedy, after reviewing an internal report about the Bay of Pigs fiasco, tore it to pieces and tossed it into the air, promising that he would "splinter the CIA in a thousand pieces and scatter it to the winds." Sure, he wished he could have done that to the CIA. Unfortunately, the CIA did it to him first. And even 57 years later, the case is too damned big and nefarious for the CIA to ever allow us to learn the whole truth about it.

I'll tell you another thing: JFK was not killed by the Mafia. They wouldn't have had the balls to knock off a sitting President. In any case, the "Mob" knew that Robert Kennedy, an aggressive Attorney General, was a much bigger threat to them when it came to conducting their business. Why would organized crime want to kill John Kennedy?

That would have left them to face the wrath of Bobby, unchecked. Plus, people within the realm of organized crime are notorious for their inability to keep secrets. The details would have come out in time. Remember Joe Valachi?

On matters and opinions related to the case of JFK, I have had some opposition, even among my colleagues. Alan Dershowitz admits that the Warren Commission investigation was sloppy and far from perfect but, nonetheless, does not argue with the conclusion that Oswald was the lone gunman. He says experience has taught him that the simplest answer is usually the right one.

F. Lee Bailey believes that the trail to President Kennedy's assassin leads directly to Cuba, where Oswald had ties. He contends that law enforcement told this to Lyndon Johnson who, as Vice President, assumed the Presidency in the aftermath of the assassination. "But," they told him, according to Lee Bailey, "If the trail leads to Castro, the American people will demand that we go in and get him."

At that time, a U.S. invasion of Cuba, regardless of the reason, would have violated the secret deal that was sealed by President Kennedy with Soviet Premier Nikita Khrushchev to end 1962's Cuban Missile Crisis. According to Lee Bailey, any such violation could have triggered another world war. And he went a step further. According to Lee, President Johnson reportedly approached Earl Warren, Chief Justice of the U.S. Supreme Court, and said something to this effect: "I'm going to appoint you to head a commission but, let me tell you what *cannot* happen: this *cannot* be connected to Cuba."

F. Lee Bailey: *[The Warren Commission] conducted a poor investigation with a faulty conclusion saying that Oswald acted alone. Few people in the business of homicide—cops, defense lawyers, and so on—think that all of those bullets and injuries were caused by a mail-order rifle by one guy who was positioned on the sixth floor of the Texas School Book Depository. That's where Cyril nailed it early on. The track of the bullet [that hit both Kennedy and Connally] is the kind of issue for which Cyril is a true expert, and it was incompatible with the Oswald scenario.*

Happy as I am to accept kudos from one of America's great attorneys, I do not agree with Lee Bailey's take on the matter. It wasn't the Cubans, the Russians or the Mafia who killed President Kennedy. It was us. If that assassination took place anywhere else in the world, we would have accepted it as just another coup. But we were unwilling to accept that such a thing could happen in America.

For the next few years, as I went about my business developing my professional career in Pittsburgh, I continued my research into the JFK case whenever time allowed. Then in the fall of 1968, I was contacted by Jim Garrison, the now legendary (and often unfairly ridiculed) District Attorney of Orleans Parish, Louisiana, who had worked feverishly to try to put together the pieces of the plot to assassinate President Kennedy.

At the time, Garrison was preparing for the trial of Clay Shaw, a New Orleans businessman who would hold the distinction of being the only person ever prosecuted in connection with the assassination of John F. Kennedy. Garrison contended that Shaw and a group of right-wing activists were involved in a conspiracy with elements of the CIA to kill the President. That group included a former FBI operative named Guy Banister, and David Ferrie, who was in the Civil Air Patrol at the same time as Lee Harvey Oswald. (Some people believe that Ferrie and Oswald met each other then, but no one knows for sure.)

I was called to testify before federal Judge Charles A. Halleck, Jr., as part of Garrison's petition for access to the autopsy materials in the Kennedy case. Those materials, unbelievably, had been sealed by order of a cockamamie document that the Feds drafted indicating that all materials related to the assassination of the President were the personal property of Mrs. Kennedy, which included the blood-spattered pink suit that she was wearing on the day of the assassination, the autopsy report and its accompanying photos and x-rays, among other items.

I often joke about that order because its directive was so patently absurd. Jackie Kennedy was probably the last person in the world who would have wanted to keep any of those things. But the federal government, in 1966, had all the materials related to the President's autopsy placed in what is called a "constructive trust," thus making the materials the rightful private property of the Kennedy family. In turn, Jackie, by way of a "memorandum of transfer," ceded the materials back to the federal government with the proviso that nobody could have access to them for 75 years—with the exception of a "qualified expert in the field of pathology with a serious historical purpose or interest," who could apply for access after five years had passed.

With the Shaw trial looming, I told Jim Garrison that to be effective on the witness stand, it was imperative that I be able to examine the autopsy evidence that was in the hands of the government. So, the DA filed a motion and again went before Judge Halleck, who ruled from the bench that the government must make all the evidence in the case of John F. Kennedy available to the prosecution. However, the Feds boldly, blatantly and disrespectfully said, in essence, that they would appeal his ruling "until hell freezes over." Clearly, they were going to fight the release of this evidentiary material to the end of the line.

In the meantime, Garrison had everything set to proceed with the trial of Clay Shaw, but the Feds and the big-shot news people were lined up against him. Access to the autopsy materials ultimately was not granted in time for the trial and, to this day, I am proud of the fact that I didn't testify in the case. I'm glad that I didn't go down to New Orleans and shoot my mouth off without having seen the autopsy materials. And I'm pleased that I had enough moral and ethical strength, and a strong enough sense of professional responsibility, to resist the temptation. But I have to admit, that case was a big deal, and it would have been fantastic to be involved.

Anyway, Clay Shaw's trial took place in January and February of 1969. Not surprisingly, he was acquitted, leaving Jim Garrison's reputation in tatters, thanks in large measure to the relentless barrage of criticism and ridicule heaped upon him by America's major media. As a result, the "conspiracy movement," of which Garrison was a part, slowed to a low ebb for years to come.

In my quest to unlock the riddle of the JFK assassination, my next significant move came in 1971. By that time, the five-year waiting period for Jackie Kennedy's constructive trust had expired so, as a "qualified expert in the field of pathology with a serious historical purpose or interest," I applied for permission to examine the autopsy materials.

The executor of the Kennedy trust was a man named Burke Marshall, who had been Deputy Attorney General under Robert Kennedy. It was he who had the authority to determine who would be granted access, and who wouldn't. So, I wrote to Marshall several times but received no replies. Fortuitously, Fred P. Graham, a stellar reporter for the *New York Times*, learned of my frustrations with this matter through the grapevine and called me to see if he could help.

Using the auspicious power of the press (or at least that of the vaunted *New York Times*), Graham succeeded in getting to Marshall and, as a result, I finally received a response to my missives. Marshall still tried to play games and delay but, in the end, he agreed to speak with me, but only if I would travel to New Haven, Connecticut, to discuss the matter with him in person. (Marshall was a professor at Yale Law School at the time.)

I'm sure he figured that I wouldn't make the trip, and that would have been that. Marshall, of course, did not know of my long history with that New England town or my summer connections to nearby Woodmont, where I had relatives and friends on whom I would have been happy to pay a visit on the way to and from New Haven. So, I made the trip, spoke with Burke Marshall, and was granted permission to inspect the JFK autopsy materials, thus becoming the first non-government-related forensic pathologist to be given the privilege. That was in August of 1972, nine months after I had first applied for permission, and it gave me chills to see and touch those pieces of American history.

When reviewing the materials, I compared the itemized list set forth in the April 1965 executive order with the October 1966 inventory. Lo and behold, that's when I discovered that certain materials were no longer listed. They had been in the government's possession, so nobody else could have touched them, but now the metal container which had held John Kennedy's brain in formalin was no longer on the list of contents. In addition, various photographs and microscopic tissue slides were also no longer listed. As a reward for his assistance, I gave this information to Fred Graham, who wrote an exclusive article that was published, page-one on August 24, 1972, in the *New York Times*. The President's brain was missing! Top-level professionals on U.S. Attorney General Ramsey Clark's 1968 panel knew about this, but never said a word.

In 1975, my search for the truth about the JFK assassination led to an invitation to testify before the U.S. President's Commission on CIA Activities within the United States, popularly known as the "Rockefeller Commission," after Nelson A. Rockefeller, who was Vice President under then-sitting President Gerald R. Ford. The Commission was charged with looking into accusations of espionage activities within the borders of the United States by the CIA. And while the JFK situation was not its sole focus, the assassination nonetheless became a major part of the inquiry. But at that time, no one on the panel was interested in my theories. It was "old news" to them.

GARY AGUILAR: *With the Rockefeller panel, you start to see the kind of bullshit that was pulled on Cyril. [And ever since] they have gone after him, hammer and tongs. But Cyril stands up and spits in their eyes. Cyril is a man of tremendous personal warmth, kindness and compassion, but he's also someone with staunch principles that he will not compromise. He will not lay down and die. Cyril is dedicated to what he believes is true and will defend it to the death. And he has paid a price and endured attacks that few men would be able to sustain successfully. What comes through, at least in my experience with him, is an unwillingness to suffer fools.*

The following year, I was contacted by TV journalist Geraldo Rivera, who had managed to obtain a copy of the famed Zapruder film and, in March, for the first time, it was broadcast to the nation. By way of this telecast, I was finally able to share with the public at large what I knew and thought about the assassination of President John F. Kennedy.

GERALDO RIVERA: *That was on "Good Night America," the ABC late-night program. We got our hands on a copy of the Zapruder film and, for the first time in history, we broadcast it and raised some serious questions about how our 35th President had died.*

The next stop in my crusade to shed light on the JFK mystery was the nation's capital. In 1976, the U.S. House of Representatives Select Committee on Assassinations (HSCA) was established as a bi-partisan Congressional panel for the purpose of reinvestigating the murders of the Rev. Martin Luther King, Jr., who had been gunned-down in Memphis in 1968, and the assassination of President John F. Kennedy.

RICHARD SPRAGUE: *Mark Lane suggested that I be considered for chairman of the HSCA. I said that I would, on certain conditions: That I'd be the head of the entire investigation; that I alone, had the right to hire and fire, to avoid having Congressmen push for friends or relatives to be hired; and that Congress made a commitment to providing the appropriate funding. My conditions were agreed to and I accepted.*

ROBERT TANENBAUM: *I was Deputy Chief Counsel to the assassinations committee and appointed a noted expert, Dr. Michael Baden, "Forensic Chairman." I had read and heard that Cyril had an opinion that was different from the mainstream and wanted to have him at the table, too. That's how we met. I eventually left that committee because I uncovered evidence that the members did not intend to pursue. It was extremely important, but the committee wasn't interested in searching for the truth. I told them before they hired me that I would not compromise on truth with respect to a murder case—or anything else for that matter. I wanted a thorough investigation.*

MICHAEL BADEN: *In 1978, as the Chief Medical Examiner of New York City, I was asked to be the chairman for the forensic pathology section of the HSCA. My first job was to pick the members for our section, and I chose Cyril and seven other forensic pathologists.*

So, I would be one of nine carefully chosen forensic pathologists to examine all of the autopsy materials when the time came to do so in 1978.

Tip O'Neill was Speaker of the House and, around that time, the Congressional Black Caucus had formed in Washington. Its members wanted to have an investigation into the assassination of Dr. Martin Luther King, Jr., as to whether one person was the assassin, or whether other people had been behind the killing as well. From a political standpoint, the Black Caucus was pushing the Democratic Party to have this investigation authorized by the House of Representatives. And with Jimmy Carter's run for re-election as President on the horizon, Tip had to make a decision.

> RICHARD SPRAGUE: *I was advised that Tip O'Neill wanted the full support of the Black Caucus [for President Carter's re-election]. Tip felt that to have an investigation just into the assassination of Dr. King would not come across well politically throughout the country. So, he thought, "Let's combine it with an investigation into the assassination of President Kennedy. People will be more accepting." That's why they decided to have the investigation into the two assassinations.*

There was a particular mindset going into those hearings. It's important to understand that some of my colleagues were people who worked with the federal government, and received government grants to support their work. As a result, I believe that they were determined to protect their futures at all costs. The Warren Commission Report was the government's official rendition of events and it was clear what the Feds were expecting to attain from our input.

As we reviewed the evidence we had before us, most of my colleagues explained-away things that they would not have tolerated in their own practices: missing slides and x-rays, for example. I even pointed out, having discovered it back in 1972, that, when I finally got access to the JFK autopsy materials, the President's brain was missing, and still had not been accounted for.

> RICHARD SPRAGUE: *The Committee's Chairman [Rep. Thomas N. Downing of Virginia] never told me that he was not planning to run for reelection. I only learned that he was leaving when Congressman Henry B. González of Texas took over as Chairman. From then on, it was a fight because González did not want to comply with the conditions that had been agreed to on my taking the job.*

The committee started doing some investigative work related to Dr. King's case, and even began some work on the matter of President Kennedy while Dick Sprague was still hiring people and fighting with Congress to get funding.

> RICHARD SPRAGUE: *In that fight, I learned that Chairman González was trying to get friends of his hired onto the committee. I also learned that Congress had balked at giving us the appropriate funds. Then I became subject of an attack in the* New York Times *and* Los Angeles Times, *simultaneously. The* New York Times, *which had written a favorable editorial when I was first appointed, had picked up on a defamation case that I had brought against the* Philadelphia Inquirer, *which I won and received a substantial award. They used that to [mischaracterize] where I was going with the investigation.*

One of the tools Dick Sprague wanted to use was a technique by which recordings of the spoken testimony of witnesses could be technically analyzed for truthfulness—much like a polygraph. This information was weaponized by the newspapers to paint Dick as some kind of dark figure who was going to violate witness' constitutional rights by recording them surreptitiously.

RICHARD SPRAGUE: *We never intended to do that, and we fought it out. We made it clear that we would let people know what we were going to do with the recordings. But, in any event, it was twisted and distorted. In addition, at the same time, we wanted certain documents from the CIA for the investigation we had been doing on Kennedy. The CIA would not turn them over. So, we issued subpoenas to the CIA for the documents. Then, Chairman González ordered me fired and called U.S. Marshals to remove me from my office. But, for the first time in the history of the U.S. Congress, members of a committee voted against the chairman and ordered me to stay on. This led to Mr. González's departure. Needless to say, he was angry with me.*

The fact of the matter was, Henry B. González wanted to get rid of Dick Sprague, one of the best trial attorneys in this country. I believe that González had no real interest in the investigation.

RICHARD SPRAGUE: *Congress continued to balk at funding it, too. Tip O'Neill arranged for me to speak in the well of the House, to Congress. It was becoming such a fight over me that, even though we had done some investigation into the King and Kennedy cases, I felt that my being there was becoming too much of an issue. At that stage, I just said, "I'd like to go on a vacation to Acapulco," and I resigned.*

At the time of his resignation, which was a damned shame, Dick didn't think that the HSCA had shown that the CIA had any concrete involvement with the assassination of President Kennedy. But he did see indications that the CIA had more contact with Oswald than they wanted known.

RICHARD SPRAGUE: *If you really want a true investigation of assassinations, don't use the Congress of the United States to do it. Conduct such investigations with real professionals.*

During my time on the Committee, the forensic pathology panel had the opportunity to meet and query Dr. James J. Humes, the chief pathologist who, with his colleagues Dr. J. Thornton Boswell and Dr. Pierre Finck, had conducted the autopsy on President Kennedy. For some reason, they saw to it that one committee member—yours truly—was excluded. Who was responsible for this? And who was responsible for the flip-flopping testimony of Humes and Boswell in subsequent years and, I might add, for the self-imposed exile of Pierre Finck, who never talked about the Kennedy matter again? Did all of this have anything to do with the facts? Draw your own inferences. In any case, Dr. Humes was subsequently elected President of the College of American Pathologists. Going along with "the program" has its rewards, you see.

Among the nine colleagues on the panel, the vote was eight to one in support of the Warren Commission Report and its conclusion that Lee Harvey Oswald had acted alone in the assassination of JFK. I was the lone dissenter. So, I said, "You guys are all board-certified, experienced forensic pathologists who, I would say, collectively, have conducted maybe 100,000 autopsies. And through your various offices, from your distinguished colleagues and predecessors, you may have connections to a quarter-of-a-million more. All I ask is that you bring me one bullet that has ever done what you claim this bullet did to President Kennedy and Governor Connally." That was more than 40 years ago, and I'm still waiting.

MICHAEL BADEN: *Cyril raised the issue that the President's brain had gone missing and had never been properly analyzed, which was significant because a bullet had gone through it. All of us agreed that the autopsy of President Kennedy was poorly done. Cyril also expressed his opinion that a second shooter had been involved, but we disagreed, having found no evidence of it.*

Acoustics evidence, however, was presented and led to the conclusion that more than one shooter could have been involved.

MICHAEL BADEN: *My experience in New York City was different from Cyril's in Pittsburgh. Back then, in New York, we had 2,200 gunshot experiences per year, so I had investigated lots and lots of gunshot wounds. But the thing that I learned from Cyril, even in times of disagreement, is that science isn't easy to follow through and people can honestly have differences of opinion.*

Some criticism of the investigation on which the Warren Commission Report was based was bandied about by the HSCA panel and those testifying, and the general opinion was that it was highly probable that some sort of conspiracy led to the assassination of the President. However, no alleged culprits were named in our final report. In fact, the Committee essentially cleared the CIA, FBI, organized crime, the Soviet Union, the anti–Castro Cuban exiles movement, and others, of being involved as a whole, while leaving open the possibility that rogue individuals from within one or more of these groups could have participated.

Ever since, no matter how hard they've tried, the Feds have not been able to convince the American public that the Warren Commission got it right. Polls conducted between 1966 and 2003 found that 60–75 percent of Americans suspected that there was a plot or a cover-up. Estimates from some polls place the numbers even higher. I'm proud of the fact that I stood there before a Congressional committee and spoke my mind.

F. LEE BAILEY: *I think my initial conversation with Cyril was about JFK, and he was dead right, and always has been about the Warren Commission. And I have special reasons to know, which I can't go into, that the "Lady in Red" was correct.*

Jean Hill, known as the "Lady in Red" because of the long, red raincoat she wore on the day of President Kennedy's assassination, was one of the witnesses closest in proximity to the President—only 21 feet away—when the historic shots were fired. She was one of several witnesses who had stated that, after the last shots were fired, she saw smoke lingering near the famed "grassy knoll" in Dealey Plaza, although this assertion does not appear in the Warren Commission Report.

F. LEE BAILEY: *The CIA and FBI were very quick to put her aside, but it was clear to me that the deadly shot came from that grassy knoll. Oswald may have fired at Kennedy [from the Texas School Book Depository], but he didn't fire the fatal shot. Cyril had all that in writing long before anyone, way before Oliver Stone made his movie.*

OLIVER STONE: *I was thinking about making "JFK" as early as 1987. I had heard the stories, but hadn't really paid attention. The editor of Jim Garrison's book was in Havana when I was there, getting an award from Fidel Castro for my film "Salvador." She cornered me in an elevator which, in socialist countries, don't usually work too well. It took about five minutes to get to the twelfth floor, and she was yapping away, "Oliver, you've just got to read this." So, I took the book from her and read it, and she was right. It was an amazing story, and I was hooked. We ran across Cyril in research and he was very authoritative. All in all, we had very good advisors for the film, and Cyril was certainly one of them, as were Jim Garrison and Fletcher Prouty [Chief of Operations for the Joint Chiefs of Staff under President Kennedy], and a number of people who were in Dallas on the day of the assassination.*

Oliver Stone visited me at my home in Squirrel Hill and asked me to consult with him on his film *JFK*. He gave me the script and, in a nice way, said, "It's been rewritten many times and we're at a point where we can't do any more rewriting." Nonetheless, he wanted me to check it for accuracy from a forensic science point-of-view. I did so, and there were a couple of errors, such as the use of the word "grams" instead of "grains" in reference to the weight or mass of the bullets that struck the President and Governor Connally, which I brought to his attention.

OLIVER STONE: *Cyril and Robert Groden were centerpieces, technically, for an analysis that something was wrong. Mark Lane picked up on it. These were civilians [who did not profit from their work]. They were doing it because something bothered them. That's called "passion." They were the earliest whistleblowers in my time. You didn't see many people like that. There were other whistleblowers before them, of course, but the JFK case brought to the surface some of the best instincts of the American people: righteous anger and a desire to see justice done.*

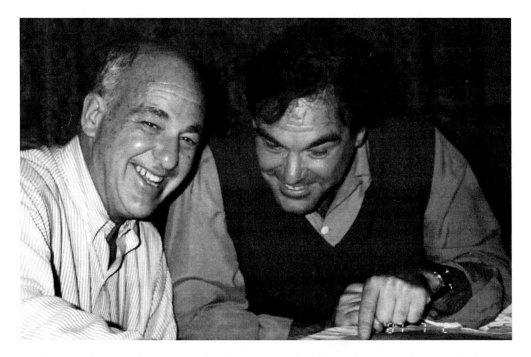

With movie director Oliver Stone after the release of his film *JFK*, on which I consulted, 1991.

During the film's production, I traveled to New Orleans to the closed courthouse which served as the set for several key scenes. Suddenly, there I was, standing back, watching hesitantly, a scene that was reported to have taken place in Jim Garrison's office. Kevin Costner, as Garrison, was seated at a desk questioning actor Joe Pesci, who was portraying possible suspect David Ferrie. The two characters ended up talking about a goose-hunting trip that Ferrie had concocted as an alibi for being in the Dallas area at the time of the assassination. The fact that David Ferrie didn't have a gun with him on the trip in question didn't matter in the least to him, but it mattered to Garrison. His story was so absurd that the actors couldn't keep straight faces and had to do the scene four or five times to get it right. When shooting was complete that morning, everyone broke for lunch and Stone called Kevin Costner over to meet me. I couldn't wait to say, "Mr. Costner, my wife adores you" but, before I could say anything to him, he reached out to shake my hand and said, "So, you're the guy that wrote all that stuff about JFK."

While on the movie set, at one point, I performed for Oliver, Kevin Costner and Joe Pesci the demonstration that I had been doing and continue to do every time I talk about JFK and the single-bullet theory, wherein I grab two people from the audience and place them in chairs: one in the rear as President Kennedy; the other in front as Governor John Connally; then I demonstrate the path that the single bullet had to have taken according to the Warren Commission. I never fail to get laughs with this because the theory is so preposterous.

DAWNA KAUFMANN: *Cyril's passion for the JFK case is formidable and crops up in unexpected ways. I've seen him stopped in restaurants and questioned about the single-bullet theory and the idea is quickly extinguished by Cyril, who will seat two people in the same positions that Kennedy and Connally were in when the shots were fired, and demonstrate the faux and factual trajectories of the bullets. Anyone who experiences this show-and-tell is instantly relieved of the "Oswald acted alone" fantasy and comes to understand the brazenly bogus attempt to cover up the historical truth. Cyril has an inexhaustible need to share this experiment and, if it takes him the rest of his life to convince one person of this, he'll consider it time well-spent.*

TONY NORMAN: *My church on the South Side [of Pittsburgh] used to have a panel once-a-month for which we would invite local luminaries to come and converse with us. One time, Cyril was nice enough to come and speak to an assembly of about 100 people. At some point, the Warren Commission came up, and I said, "This is where you and I part company, Cyril, because I'm much less conspiratorial than you." I think that there is a rational explanation for what happened that day and I don't think that it involved large machinations.*

I said that I believe that Lee Harvey Oswald—whether he acted alone in the cosmic sense or not—certainly pulled the trigger, and Cyril, without missing a beat, stepped off the podium and asked two people who were sitting in the front row to stand up. He took their chairs, moved them out and said to those two people, "You are going to be John F. Kennedy; and you are going to be John Connally." He then proceeded to provide details about how fast the car was going, and so on, after which he hopped back up on stage and said, "I'm Lee Harvey Oswald." Cyril then mimicked having a gun in his hands and pro-

ceeded to "shoot" saying, "This is the trajectory of the bullet." Next, he left the stage again and went down to the audience to show the bullet's impact as it traveled through two bodies, twisting, turning, and so on, after which he said to the congregation, as if he were ending an argument for a jury, "If you're good Christians, it wouldn't surprise me if you believe the single-bullet theory, because to do so would take a leap of faith." And he had the congregation howling and applauding wildly.

My demonstration in New Orleans must have gone over well because Oliver put it in his movie. Kevin Costner, as DA Jim Garrison, makes that very presentation at the Clay Shaw trial to show the absurdity of the single-bullet theory. That was my major contribution to Oliver's movie, *JFK.*

OLIVER STONE: *Cyril was obviously qualified. We did a great autopsy scene with his help. And he gave me some solid ideas in the courtroom, too. He helped me stage the evidence scene, which I had not seen Garrison do because Garrison was an old man when we worked on the movie.*

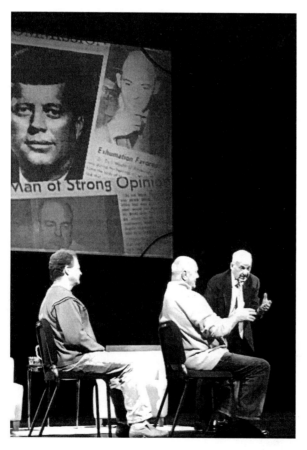

A live demonstration of the Warren Commission's "single-bullet theory." When I did this for director Oliver Stone, he elected to have Kevin Costner perform the same routine in Stone's blockbuster movie *JFK.*

At the outset of the film, a quote appears on a black screen from American author and poet Ella Wheeler Cox: "To sin by silence when we should protest makes cowards out of men." I'm glad that I've stayed on the case and have never "fell silent." I will be on the case until the end.

OLIVER STONE: *I respect Cyril enormously because he's stayed out there in the public eye and has continued to say what he believes. He's a straight shooter. I remember him vividly as one of the "good guys" who supported us. He was clear and persuasive and I believed him entirely. I saw Cyril in Pittsburgh [at Duquesne University] for an event to mark the 50th anniversary of the Kennedy assassination. He looked the same, exactly, as he did years ago, when I first met him. I said to him, "What happened, Cyril? Do you take formaldehyde with your cereal? You're preserving yourself so well." He just laughed and said, "Just some Hgb and a steroid mix."*

When it came to my investigative work and controversial public statements regarding the JFK assassination, my wife admits to having been more than a bit concerned at first.

SIGRID WECHT: *In the early days, Cyril would have people stay at our house all the time. I was busy with the kids and didn't have time to worry too much about it but, as time went on, I became more and more concerned about his involvement with the Kennedy case. We've all heard about people who have been killed in pursuit of the truth. In fact, one gentleman, a Dutchman, came to our home to interview Cyril and warned that, if Cyril looked into this too much, something bad might very well happen to him.*

Admittedly, in the early years of my investigation, I often allowed fellow truth-seekers, such as the aforementioned Dutchman, to stay at our home. To Sigrid, the Wecht household became a makeshift crossroads for the JFK investigation and its attendant horde of conspiracy buffs.

SIGRID WECHT: *The kids got used to seeing strange people—Americans, Europeans, Africans and Asians—around the house. Now and then, some opportunistic fakers came and latched on to Cyril, like the couple who claimed that they knew where John Kennedy's missing brain was located and would lead Cyril to it. These kinds of people came and went all the time.*

Sigrid is thankful, however, that I have largely been able to cut through the nonsense, to weed out opportunists and phonies.

SIGRID WECHT: *Cyril flirts with their ideas sometimes, but he has a very good mind, and doesn't allow himself to be misled by some of the schmendricks ["stupid people," in Yiddish] who show up at the various JFK conferences. You can just smell them coming.*

DAVID WECHT: *Some guy once insisted on meeting with my dad. He said that he had the secret to the Kennedy assassination, so my dad met with him, and brought my brother, Ben. This guy showed them a segment of the Zapruder film and began freezing, blowing up and zooming in to particular frames, which were all pixelated. He kept saying, "Do you see that?" Ben and my dad said, "No." So, he took a grease pen out and circled an opaque area. "We still don't see anything. What is it?" to which the man responded, "That's the head of the achondroplastic dwarf who was in the limo and firing at President Kennedy."*

And Sigrid, as brave and vocal as I am, would, at times, express doubts when she had them about some of my notions about the assassination of JFK and the ideas of others.

SIGRID WECHT: *He gets mad at me when I do that because he gives everyone a chance. That's the kind of person he is. It's probably the Norwegian in me that makes me skeptical and suspicious. I often have my doubts about people, but Cyril is trusting and polite. He is a great communicator, and he loves to converse and schmooze, even with nuts. I wonder if we'll see any results from all of his efforts regarding this JFK business. I know it's important but, sometimes, I feel that going over and over this Kennedy thing is like beating a dead horse.*

In my estimation, from the day of the assassination, the news media establishment began lapping up what the federal government was feeding them and have never really stopped. Remember, this was pre–Vietnam and pre–Watergate. When the government spoke, the media listened. They bought in and stuck with it. It's an albatross around their necks, one of the greatest failures in their collective history.

For people like Dan Rather and Peter Jennings, their careers and reputations bloomed and blossomed as a result of their coverage in those years, and they weren't about to back off from what they'd said. They were egocentric people to the ultimate degree. But remember, 60–75 percent of Americans continue to reject the Warren Commission's conclusions. Is that hard science? No. But tell me how many issues in American politics consistently, over decades, have two-thirds or three-fourths of the public voting the same way? Why can't we allow it to go away? Don't many murders go unsolved? Sure, they do. But not murders of American Presidents.

My adversarial attitude toward government—and, at times, the press—is what has always made me appear dangerous to the establishment (and sometimes to myself). In my opinion, the level of paranoia in America knows no bounds, and this includes the criminal justice system and the corporate media. It reaches a point at which they must protect their own reputations and images. When you're a professional person considering the murder of a sitting President—I'm talking about my colleagues in forensic science and the people in the press—and you chose to stand by the official government version of events, how can you reverse that later on, even when new evidence accrues against it? You can't. You're stuck, and so they are.

I have been reiterating my views about the JFK case for more than 50 years, which is much akin to banging one's head on concrete because what I believe and have been espousing likely will never be proven. But had that horrible event happened in this era of high-technology, I believe that the media would have pounced on the story like famished hyenas. Imagine the number of cell phones that would have captured still photographs and videos of the Presidential motorcade, from a dizzying array of distinct vantage points, and with image clarity unattainable in the early 1960s. Or how about the drumbeat of blanket, round-the-clock news coverage on cable, not to mention the vast number of uncensored theories that would no doubt be pinging around the blogosphere? The Feds wouldn't be able to control something like the Kennedy assassination if it happened today. Put it all together: a passive public, ambivalent criminal justice professionals and legislators, and gutlessness on the part of our major news media. How could they all just accept what was being told to them without a struggle?

The government took advantage of our collective shock as a nation. In the past, the media knew things but we never learned about them, such as mistresses in the White House. It's true that the media "safety net" for government officials was ultimately torn by the truths revealed about the Vietnam War and the Watergate scandal, and finally fell through under the weight of Bill Clinton and Monica Lewinsky. Today's news media may have reached a new level of obnoxiousness, but it's a different world today, especially for the rich and powerful. Nothing will stay secret for long.

The *coup d'état* that left President Kennedy dead may not be proven by me, Oliver Stone or anyone else, but I believe that the truth is out there. I don't know if anybody knows the names of all the individuals involved, but the perpetrators had to be people who were extremely knowledgeable and experienced—experts, really—in this kind of clandestine activity; people who knew the way the game is played and had the power to make the appropriate contacts to set things in motion and carry out their mission. To whom does that bring us? It brings us to the people who do "spook" operations. It brings us to people involved in the CIA, which has splinter groups that are not recognized officially except by one or two people who are in the know.

I don't believe that the people in charge of the CIA at that time planned and carried out the assassination of John F. Kennedy. I believe that the culprits were people who had CIA connections, who had those kinds of contacts, that kind of knowledge and expertise, that kind of power, and who also, politically, had the motivation, the desire, the need to act. When these people see the flag flying, it's different for them than it is for the average American. Some people keep a secret better than others. It's a matter of inculcated philosophy and rigid training over years. When you're talking about these organizations, secrecy is their religion. These are ideological "true believers." They will take their secrets to the grave.

If you're a true believer in a specific vision of America, and you see your country going down the tubes with John Kennedy "bowing and scraping" to the Russians, failing to make a decisive move against Castro, and failing to do what was necessary to win in Vietnam, what do you do? These are the same people who wanted us to drop atomic bombs on Russia at the close of World War II. The only way to save the country was a coup. And not everything was planned. Some things just fell into place.

Today, we're still learning about things that our government did in World War II, Korea and Vietnam. Not that they are unimportant, but compared to the assassination of a sitting President, they pale by comparison. If the government could cover up some things about what we did in wars a half-century ago—an execution we allowed, or a village we wiped out—why couldn't it cover up the truth about the assassination of a U.S. President?

All in all, the JFK assassination case was a real eye-opener for me. Given my personality, my political philosophy, and my attitude toward arrogant, militant, dictatorial people in government, my disgust probably would have bubbled to the surface eventually. There's no question that what was instilled in me by the JFK case may have already been there lying dormant, eventually to be expressed. But this happened sooner than it might have when, through my JFK investigation, I became aware of how governmental agencies and top-notch people can lie, manipulate, scheme and deceive. I'm sure that, no matter what, the assassination and its aftermath certainly exacerbated, catalyzed, and accentuated my strong feelings of disdain and outright rejection and hostility toward certain kinds of actions taken by our government.

For years following my discharge from the Air Force in 1961, I was friendly with the personnel at the Armed Forces Institute of Pathology, and I lectured there. After I got caught up in the pursuit of truth regarding the assassination of President John F. Kennedy in the 1970s, I was never again invited to lecture at programs that the organization put on, despite the fact that I was President of the American Academy of Forensic Sciences. Similarly, although I lectured by invitation at the FBI Academy, over time,

I stopped receiving invitations there, too. It seemed that, the more I spoke out about the JFK assassination, the less I was asked to participate in programs at various professional organizations that have national committees. The College of American Pathologists and the American Society of Clinical Pathologists never invited me to sit on any of their forensic pathology committees. I'm not suggesting that this was organized in some kind of a grand schematic fashion. But an attitude, a feeling, was communicated: "We don't want Wecht. Even if he comes here talking about some other subject, people will ask him about JFK," and they didn't want that. How much of this has been directly and solely related to my stance vis-à-vis JFK, and how much of it may have been related to the fact that I have spoken out on any number of other controversial matters, I can't say.

> DAVID WECHT: *I don't remember the context and details, but I do remember, at one point, that a lawyer on my dad's behalf made a Freedom of Information Act (FOIA) request [for government records pertaining to "Cyril H. Wecht"] and he got back a bunch of stuff that was heavily redacted. The federal government often claims all sorts of enumerated exceptions to the FOIA. But even though those records were blacked-out, it was clear that J. Edgar Hoover and his successors had been keeping tabs on my dad because he has always fought the power.*

Without question, the story of JFK bothers me a lot still, as does the tale of RFK. Interestingly, while so much emphasis has been placed on the case of John Kennedy—which is understandable because he was, after all, President of the United States—in my estimation, the case of Robert Kennedy is a more obvious travesty. The Robert F. Kennedy case, if it had been handled properly, would have reached a totally different conclusion. The case regarding RFK was even more unequivocally absurd than JFK's. Let me get right to the heart of it. Robert Kennedy had just won the California primary. To get the candidate through the cheering crowd at the Ambassador Hotel would have taken hours, so it was decided to take Senator Kennedy out another way, through the kitchen, where it's said that Sirhan Sirhan shot at him as he approached.

Over the past 50 years or so, I've talked about the RFK assassination to many thousands of people, if you put all of my audiences together. Every time, no matter who is in the audience, I ask, especially when some older people are in attendance who were actually alive at the time and can recall the assassination: "From what distance would you say the kill shot was fired?"

The answers to this question over the years have been many. Some say "six feet"; some, "eight feet"; others say "10 feet"; and so on. When I tell them that the actual distance from which the shot that killed Bobby Kennedy was fired was from one- to one-and-one-half inches away, striking him behind the right ear, I hear gasps. This is not an opinion; it is a scientific conclusion. My old friend, Dr. Tom Noguchi, did the autopsy on RFK, with six board-certified forensic pathologists on his staff, three board-certified military forensic pathologists, three civilian forensic pathologists who were called in as official consultants, Dr. William Eckert, Dr. Russell Fisher (both now deceased), and me. We all concurred that the shot was fired from one- to one-and-one-half inches away. Dr. Noguchi reported this in his testimony to the grand jury when asked, but at the trial of Sirhan, the subject was never raised, not by the prosecution, obviously, nor by the defense. Tom has never backed away from the fact, though he hasn't chosen to broadcast it widely either.

The only forensic expert called upon by Sirhan's defense was a forensic psychiatrist, to talk about whether or not Sirhan suffered from diminished capacity under California state law. This was to lay the groundwork for an "insanity plea," which is the way we refer to it, generically. But excluding this psychiatrist, Grant Cooper, an experienced defense attorney, never consulted a forensic science expert, criminalist or ballistics expert, and never cross-examined Tom Noguchi about the shots, the distance from which they were fired, the trajectory, and so on.

There are other problems with the RFK case, too, such as the number of shots fired. An investigation led to the conclusion that there were 13. But Sirhan's gun held only eight bullets. He shot them all, firing wildly, and he sure as hell never reloaded. (Five people were hit and survived.) RFK was hit four times. And as I've said, the fatal shot hit him behind his right ear. All four shots that hit Bobby Kennedy were fired from behind him, at a distance of no more than six inches. Nobody has ever placed Sirhan's gun that close to the Senator. The headshot was likely first, followed by the others as he sank to the floor.

Bullet holes in the kitchen's door frames were ignored initially and, when investigators went back to revisit them, they were gone. A gun belonging to Thane Eugene Cesar, a freelance security guard that evening, who was directly behind and to the right of Senator Kennedy, was never taken and tested. Months later, when investigators went back to retrieve Mr. Cesar's gun, they learned that he had sold it. They then traced the sale, finally, to a man in Arkansas. When asked if he had indeed purchased the gun, the man said "Yes." "Then where is the gun, sir?" "Well, it was in my second-floor bedroom, but it was stolen."

While we cannot know everything precisely, Sirhan was, at the least, guilty of the attempted murder of the five other people who were hit by bullets on that June night in California. And he may have been involved in a conspiracy to kill Bobby, even though there is good reason to believe that he was hypno-programmed to commit this act. Sirhan has no memory of what happened, so he can't express remorse, which is why his appeals are always denied. And Thane Eugene Cesar was never charged for any crime that occurred that night; he died in 2019.

The fact that the bullet that killed Bobby Kennedy hit him behind his right ear from a distance of no more than one-and-one-half inches never came out at Sirhan's trial, and there will never be a retrial. Whether or not it was a set-up, or if it was an accidental shooting by a security guard who was standing near Robert Kennedy, no one can really say. But again, I saw injustice, especially in the face of scientific proof. All the defense wanted to do was to "prove" that Sirhan was insane. Incidentally, in the fall of 1968, Sirhan's mother called me out of the blue to ask if I would be her son's lawyer. I was tempted, but decided that I was too busy with my forensic pathology work and my young family to devote the time needed to provide adequate legal counsel. Furthermore, I was not an experienced criminal trial attorney.

In my younger days, I didn't think such things could happen. But there are certain cases and particular issues that are not going to be resurrected. They are "too hot to handle" and the facts will remain buried for a long time, if not forever. With government cover-ups, the public has, I suppose, come to accept that we have little choice but to let things be. The Feds can't ever allow the American people to know that high-level political assassinations have occurred and could occur again anytime in the good old U.S.A.

I believe that national nightmares such as the assassinations of John and Robert Kennedy aren't always highly organized affairs. Some seem to arrive *sui generis*. Things erupt because they must. You can count on it. So, I see all of these horrible things, and then witness the arrogance, naiveté and ignorance, speaking broadly, of the American public. Bad guys in nice suits are still bad guys, and they kill kings, prime ministers and presidents in other countries. Why not in the U.S.?

ALEC BALDWIN: *I have seen Dr. Wecht's name connected to the JFK case for many years and, lately, I have followed the conferences that he hosts at Duquesne University. He is an old warrior, someone who has fought hard to keep the issue of the Warren Commission's conclusions alive in academia and in the media.*

Alec Baldwin, star of stage, screen and television, played my colleague, Dr. Julian Bailes, in the Hollywood movie *Concussion*. Released in 2015, the film focused on pathologist Dr. Bennet Omalu—who worked for me—and the truth about brain damage in football players. (The part of "Dr. Cyril Wecht" was played by actor Albert Brooks.)

ALEC BALDWIN: *When I had dinner with him not too long ago, I could still see bright flashes of the curiosity, the indignation, and the fire that have propelled his legendary career for five decades.*

So, the plans for the assassination of President John F. Kennedy did not emanate or spring from the malevolent minds of people in Moscow or Havana, or from the meeting rooms of the Mob. Well-placed Americans were behind this, and that's very painful, indeed. Think about J. Edgar Hoover and Lyndon Johnson. Were there two more politically-savvy and powerful individuals in America at that time? Was there anything that, if they wanted to find out, they could not have found out? I don't believe that Hoover or Johnson had anything to do with the primary conspiracy to kill John Kennedy. But do I believe that they came to know everything later on? You bet. Who knows who all was responsible? My purpose has always been to seek truth and justice, and to come to know and recognize what happened on November 22, 1963.

As a nation, had we five more years led by Jack and eight years after that led by Bobby, what might have happened? Would there have been a warming with Russia? What about détente with Cuba? Would we have withdrawn from Vietnam? The point is, some positive things might have happened over the ensuing 13 years. But there was no way in the world that that was going to be allowed. There was only one way to bring back the kind of America that the assassins believed should exist. They were not going to let the U.S. go down that winding, "treacherous" road on which Jack Kennedy and his brother Bobby were leading us. The assassination of the President was the overthrow of the government. It was a *coup d'etat*. That's what happened in America.

> ALEC BALDWIN: *The unsettled nature of the [John F. Kennedy assassination] case is beyond significant in American life. The fact that we have not adequately embraced the truth about who was responsible for this is one thing that accounts for America's decline since the 1960s.*

As the years have passed, I have received calls about the deaths of Elvis Presley, JonBenét Ramsey, Laci Peterson, and many others. But make no mistake: all of my high-profile consultations, starting with my work regarding the case of RFK with Tom Noguchi, likely would never have come about if not for my passion for, and obsession with, the assassination of President John F. Kennedy.

Many years ago, I established correspondence with Lee Harvey Oswald's widow, Marina, through a mysterious man named George Sergius de Mohrenschildt, a petroleum geologist and professor who had befriended the Oswalds in the summer of 1962, when they moved to Texas. He maintained that friendship until Oswald's death, two days after the JFK assassination.

George de Mohrenschildt was a Russian, post–Revolution émigré to the U.S. He

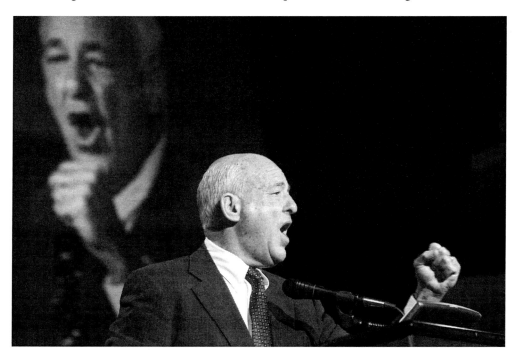

Raising the roof at a commemorative conference marking the 40th anniversary of JFK's assassination, sponsored by the Cyril H. Wecht Institute of Forensic Science and Law at Duquesne University, 2003 (*Pittsburgh Post-Gazette*).

and his family fled Russia over the business with the Bolsheviks after World War I. He was not independently wealthy, but he was tied to some big oil interests and worked with several American oil barons.

In March of 1977, de Mohrenschildt received a business card from an investigator for the House Select Committee on Assassinations saying that he would like to meet with him that afternoon, after which de Mohrenschildt committed suicide.

I once went to de Mohrenschildt's apartment in Dallas and met with him and his wife. That was the opening to Marina. She and I corresponded and, soon, talked on the telephone. Then we set up a meeting and had lunch with her, in the Dallas area, which was very pleasant. We got along quite well. That meeting established a relationship that has continued through the years, even to the present time. She, I think, trusts me. Marina, understandably, won't talk to many people. Imagine how she has been bothered over the years. She probably has had thousands of contacts.

I have talked with Marina about her relationship with Lee and his feelings and thoughts, and whether he had ever expressed animosity toward JFK, personally or politically, and the answers to such questions have always been "No." Marina was quite firm in her belief that her husband, Lee Harvey Oswald, did not assassinate John F. Kennedy and, in fact, had played no role in it.

I have been speaking about the JFK assassination for decades, on TV and in the press, and at many venues including the Cyril H. Wecht Institute of Forensic Science and Law, and at conferences sponsored by Citizens Against Political Assassinations (CAPA), an organization for which I am Chairman. Through CAPA, my colleagues and I remain in pursuit of the release of withheld records related to the assassination. Our goal is to find the truth, once and for all, and to seek justice.

Media Darling

Sometimes I'm praised and at times I'm mocked for being a "media darling," one of those colorful and quotable people whose commentary makes television and radio programs more interesting and entertaining. I may be that, to some degree, but I assure you that I am no "media whore," a person who needs to promote himself shamelessly for the sole purpose of self-aggrandizement.

JOHN MCINTIRE: *When I first came to town, I couldn't get a Pittsburgher to do my show, literally. Nobody knew who I was and nobody wanted to get involved with me, except the brave and fearless Cyril Wecht. I was fascinated by him. He was the easiest guest to host because you could ask him a question and, a full 15 minutes later, you could ask him a second. I was mesmerized by the rhythm of his speech. He's an amazing communicator, and a real character.*

JOSEPH MAROON: *Very early on in my career, I became aware of Cyril's incredible vocabulary and his ability to articulate things better than almost anyone I'd ever heard.*

CHRIS MOORE: *Most of my history with Cyril is through on-air programs and interviews. By now, I would call him a friend. I like interviewing Cyril because he just has so much to say. We have fun every time we talk. The folks in the control room at the station always joke with me, saying, "All you have to do is ask one question, and we'll wake you up in an hour."*

JOHN MCINTIRE: *Cyril doesn't need any local media "dweebs" like myself, yet he'll work with us and, if things go well, he'll befriend us. There's not much in it for him, but he does it anyway. He even shows up for the cabaret shows I do. At 10:30 on certain Saturday nights, he'll come out and goof around with me on stage for 50 or 60 people—if we're lucky. And he always says things like, "How can we get more people here?" He wants a large audience, always.*

I've been giving media interviews going back as far as the late 1960s, yet I've never had an agent, not for my media or public appearances, nor for my books. I don't have anyone promoting me. And I don't contact people myself. They contact me. Why? It's called "credibility." I call things as I see them, no matter the situation or who is involved. Media-types like that about me.

KATHY McCABE: *People from the news media never stop calling him. Anytime there is a high-profile case in the news, they call. They all want his take on things. He's been on all of the network and cable shows, and lots of radio shows, too. His knowledge and energy are amazing.*

I'm not one to tell colleagues in my field to engage the media as much as I do. That's entirely up to them. But if any of them who, because of their passivity, shyness or arrogance, believe that I appear in the media too often, screw them. With the exception of maybe a half-dozen times in my 50 years of granting media interviews, I have not been paid to appear on TV, on radio, or in the press. I don't do it for the money. I do it to be involved, and to try to bring some sense to complicated situations. My family will attest to the fact that, after any media appearance, no matter who it was with or what the subject was, I never tune in to see or hear myself afterward. I haven't the time for it. I may read newspaper stories in which I've been quoted, but that comes about naturally, during my daily review of local and national events.

Today in Pittsburgh, the media is a "toothless tiger." The reporters here are so timid, fearful that they might lose their jobs, I suppose, as the stars in the media firmament shift unpredictably above their heads. But it wasn't always so. The city used to have some solid journalists, some real "ball-breakers," who were not always friendly to me. But I respected their spirit and desire to get their jobs done. Andy Sheehan, before he left the *Pittsburgh Post-Gazette* for KDKA-TV, was one. Andrew Schneider was another, from the *Pittsburgh Press*, who won Pulitzer Prizes in 1986 and 1987. So, where have all the investigative reporters gone? Don't tell me "to the blogosphere." The truth is that most news organizations, whether in print, broadcast or even online, can't afford or refuse to pay for investigative reporting anymore, and we're all the worse for it.

Anyway, what I do with my time is my business. I'm my own person. I do what I want, and try to fit as many things into my schedule as possible, media appearances included. I enjoy engaging and sometimes doing battle with the media. I find it challenging and, I believe, I'm good at it. Sometimes colleagues will remark snidely that they saw me on *Geraldo*, on *Larry King Live* or, more recently, on *Dr. Phil*, as if I'd done something untoward. Trust me, they would all love to be doing it, too, but haven't the talent, nor have they put in the time and effort to make themselves known. But wrangling with the media, while often fun, can be fraught with peril, too.

A brief recap of a period in my professional history will help to frame what comes next. In 1956–57, I served a one-year internship at St. Francis Hospital in Pittsburgh. Then, from 1957 to 1959, I did two years of residency in anatomic and clinical pathology at the University of Pittsburgh Veterans Administration Hospital—and also attended two years of law school at Pitt. From 1959–61, I served a two-year hitch in U.S. Air Force, where I was a Captain and Associate Pathologist at Maxwell Air Force Base in Montgomery, Alabama. During my obligatory military service, I received credit for two years of further training in pathology.

Once discharged from the Air Force, I accepted a forensic pathology fellowship in Baltimore. I was Associate Pathologist and Research Fellow in Forensic Pathology at the Office of the Chief Medical Examiner of Maryland, and finished my third year of law school in the evenings at the University of Maryland. For a little extra money, I also served as the pathologist for a small hospital in Baltimore. Then, in 1962, I returned to Pittsburgh for good, a bona fide forensic pathologist bound for private practice. It was at this time that I was invited to be a member of the Allegheny County Medical Society's "Committee for the Medical Examiner System."

Naturally, I became the Committee's most vocal spokesperson, repeating the catchphrase for our efforts for dramatic effect: "You can get away with murder in Allegheny County," which, as you know, incensed City of Pittsburgh homicide chief Eugene Coon, who felt that I was attacking him personally, which was not my intention. I was simply referring to the failure of the Allegheny County Coroner's Office (that one day I would lead) to conduct autopsies or to add a forensic pathologist to its staff.

Gene Coon was well-connected with the news media back then. Reporters always want a connection with the head of homicide to get hot tips on murder stories. As mentioned previously, one day, I picked up the *Pittsburgh Press* and read a front-page story attacking me for the way I was allegedly portraying Coon, who was quoted throughout. But the reporter never contacted me for rebuttal. That's when I came to learn that journalists don't always do a good job of presenting issues. My troubles with the Pittsburgh media started off in that fashion. Now, let's jump to 1979.

It was in or around April and, even though I'd been indicted in my first go-around with accusations of "public corruption," I was endorsed by the Allegheny County Democratic Committee to run for County Commissioner with Tom Foerster. Commissioner Leonard Staisey had been elected to the Court of Common Pleas, so Tom asked me to fill the bill and run with him. Foerster, however, who had been around forever in local politics, told me that, shortly thereafter, he received a personal visit at his office from Leo Koeberlein, managing editor of the *Pittsburgh Press*.

Koeberlein was a major player in the city at that time and a very strong personality. He urged Foerster to drop me as his running mate. Tom told me that, in all the years he had been involved in politics, Koeberlein never called him, not even once. I'll tell you this, right now: That visit, I believe, was prompted by anti–Semitism. What other reason would Koeberlein have had to try to force me out? If he had written an editorial, fine. That's different. But a personal, private visit?

Needless to say, Koeberlein hammered me with negative coverage in the *Press* that was horribly one-sided. (This happened at the *Post-Gazette* also, but to a lesser extent.) That set the stage for a poor relationship with the paper from then on. Shirley Uhl, who was a news reporter there at the time, was a nice and knowledgeable guy. I tried, in later years, after Shirley left *The Press*, to learn from him more of the background and, perhaps, the precise reason for the animosity shown toward me from John Troan, the editor, and Leo Koeberlein, but I never got a clear picture.

As for the *Post-Gazette*, I don't know all of the specifics about its long-time Editor-in-Chief, John Craig, and his personal animus, but he, too, had developed a major "hard-on" for me. Craig was a terribly unpleasant individual—egotistical, smug and intellectually ruthless. Sure, I wrote "letters to the editor" and criticized the paper sometimes, as a liberal Democrat. But I was writing to a not wildly liberal but certainly more to the "left-of-center" newspaper than the *Pittsburgh Press*, so there shouldn't have been any political bias. What in the world was going on there?

Tony Norman: *Many Pittsburghers are Roman Catholic, working-class people. A lot of folks don't have college degrees. Then in comes Cyril Wecht from the Hill District: a Jewish fighter, who's vastly more articulate than anyone within 100 miles. I do think there was a residual anti–Semitic vibe when it came to dealing with Cyril, but one could never really prove that. I know that his ongoing battle with the editorial board of the* Post-Gazette *was based upon Cyril's belief that the paper has an anti–Semitic agenda.*

When I joined the paper in 1988, John Craig was at his zenith, and his ego, power and influence in the city troubled Cyril. The interaction between Craig and Cyril really was the battle it seemed, but I thought it was crazy for the editorial board to adopt a defensive posture towards him. I thought Cyril was a fascinating character and I wanted to get to know him on my own terms, not based on whatever the history was between him and the paper's Board. I wanted to get to know him for his own merits and, to a certain extent, I did. I went on radio and TV with him, and even met him on social occasions. I got to know him by talking to him, and not just about politics, but about books. He's very literate and I appreciated that he was a public intellectual. He is a politician, a man of science, and a man of tremendous principle.

Hop Kendrick: *John Craig did not like Cyril. Once, I had to attend a meeting about something or other, so I went down to the paper, and Craig said to me, "If we're going to discuss Cyril Wecht, I'm going to walk out of here." I said, "But you invited me." He said, "Yes, but I did not invite you here to discuss your friend, Dr. Wecht. And I'm not going to let you do that to me." Nine or 10 other people were there, and they told me not to talk about Cyril because the meeting was important and they needed Craig to stay. So, I said, "OK." But Cyril is my guy. He doesn't care if you like him or not. John Craig was an arrogant bastard and Wecht wouldn't cater to him. He never catered to anybody. With Cyril Wecht, what you see is what you get.*

Rabbi Alvin Berkun: *Cyril has often taken on the* Post-Gazette. *Talk about being fearless. Here's a media source that could do him harm and, in fact, had done him some over the years, but he never cared. When he felt they were biased on issues related to Israel, or wrong with respect to whatever the issue is, he called them on it. He was not afraid of the paper or its readers.*

When it came to John Craig, challenging his newspaper was like challenging him. Attacking his paper was attacking him, personally. I once sued the *Post-Gazette* and its cartoonist, Tim Menees, over a vicious cartoon it ran about me that was more than insulting and demeaning; it was defamatory. Don't forget, you can do more damage to a person's reputation with a picture than you can with the proverbial thousand words from some pusillanimous reporter. The suit, however, was unsuccessful. When you're a public figure, to win a defamation suit is next to impossible. There's no reason for the news media or anybody to make a comment, pejorative or otherwise, about "Joe Smith," who drives a truck. The readers don't give a damn about him. Joe's irrelevant. But once you become a public figure, you have to take all kinds of bullshit from them.

I know that my outspokenness has, often enough, irritated and irked people in and beyond the media, and gave rise to some serious animosity toward me from individuals whom I have never met and who don't know anything about me, personally, and I've paid a price for it. I've lost out on things over the years because of my clashes with "authority"—appointments here and there, awards and honors, and so on. I could write a book on that subject alone. But these kinds of retributions play-out in spades when it comes to the news media because, it's one thing for "Joe Smith," a private citizen, or even somebody in the professional fields of medicine or law, to dislike me. But reporters possess the power to write about me, and smear me broadly with the public.

I can understand Gene Coon being pissed off at me because of our "getting away with murder" campaign. But he knew full well that homicide investigators were often coercing confessions from people. Coon and his cohorts were not out solving murders "by the book," I'll tell you that. Now, let's look at things more precisely. Where was the media during all the years that the County Coroner's Office didn't even have a microscope? Where were they when Allegheny County, then home to 1.65 million people, didn't have a forensic pathologist doing autopsies? The first medical examiner system in the U.S. was started in Massachusetts in 1887. Where was Allegheny County? Asleep at the switch, as always.

But of all the pot-shot artists who have graced the pages of the Pittsburgh dailies, columnist Brian O'Neill of the *Post-Gazette* got under my skin the most. Don't get me started on the topic of newspaper "columnists." They all seem to think that they're authorities on everything. But when they write about something, what is their base of knowledge? What is their range of experience? Where did they acquire such great insight? When you respond to them, you're called "controversial," "outspoken," "hypersensitive," or even a "big mouth." Think about it. Does the First Amendment say that it's all right for them to speak about an issue, but not anybody else? I do not have a friendly relationship with Brian O'Neill. I have never met him in my life, except maybe once in a superficially amiable fashion, and I do not know why he has always been so hostile towards me. But just to show that I'm not unforgiving, another guy who made caustic remarks about me every now and then was Eric Heyl of the *Pittsburgh Tribune-Review*, yet he and I became quite friendly later on. Brian O'Neill is an outlier, I guess.

O'Neill, who seems to have become a writer about subjects of a totally uninteresting nature, over time, continued to take shots at me so, finally, I laid him out. He was expressing his opinions about a matter for which he was not qualified, and criticized me. I said, in essence, "Here's me, with medical and law degrees, and decades of experience. Then there's you, a young, green, local newspaper reporter," and so on. I copied all of his editors, and never heard from him after that. Behold the introductory paragraph of one of my letters to Brian O'Neill, dated May 25, 2000: *"Dear Mr. O'Neill: Smugness, ignorance of subject matter, and sycophancy are a deadly combination, especially in the person of a newspaper columnist..."*

Was that too strong? O'Neill was commenting on something of which he knew nothing: the Allegheny County Row Offices. He and his fellow *Post-Gazette* staffers were insisting that there was a need for "merit hiring" to prevent nepotism and cushy arrangements for Row Officer positions, for which they had no evidence. You would have thought that the matter was of grave concern.

Later on, in that same missive: *"...So, your May 25th column, "Roddey gets his ducks in a row," has enabled you to score some points with [John] Craig and a polyglot collection of Republicans, Wecht-haters, and various other malcontents. This will give you a perverted psychological thrill and sustain your selfish visceral needs until your next glib column..."* Well, he asked for it.

> JOHN MCINTIRE: *Brian O'Neill is the only guy I know who will dispute the fact that Cyril Wecht is brilliant. He'll say things like, "Fine, the guy is smart. And yes, it takes brains to be a doctor and a lawyer. But brilliant? Come on. That's Albert Einstein." I believe that O'Neill once wrote a column featuring quotes from letters he'd received from Cyril over the years. That did not go over well.*

It sometimes amazes me, but the treatment one receives, even when appearing via otherwise reputable national media outlets, can be just as bad. Here are some excerpts from a letter I wrote to CBS's Peter Van Sant on May 20, 2015, concerning his treatment of my commentary in a "48 Hours" TV program. I had been consulted by the Beaver County DA in a controversial homicide case, even though I had not performed the autopsy. The defendant was ultimately found guilty.

"Mr. Van Sant: ... If the objective of your program had been to disparage and attack me professionally, rather than present an overall investigative report of a case in which I was only one of many witnesses, you could not have done a better job... How is it possible that you failed to comprehend and include in your show the single most damning piece of the prosecution's case, and indeed, the key feature of my testimony? ... Incredibly, you chose to believe the explanation set forth [by the attorneys for the defendant].... Too bad for [the defense] that you were not on the jury. You might have succeeded in convincing the other eleven jurors to remove their brains from their cranial vaults while you advanced your brilliant explanation..." I received no response.

Now, I admit that, sometimes, I get caught up in the emotion of the moment, especially when the subject is Israel or the Jewish people. Gerald Schiller of Penn Hills was the recipient of a personal letter from me in response to his "letter to the editor" that appeared in the *Post-Gazette* on January 27, 2014. In it, Schiller expressed support for the views of former U.S. Ambassador Daniel H. Simpson, who had accused the Israelis of fomenting war between Sunni and Shiite Muslims. My letter, dated January 28, left no doubt about my opinion regarding Schiller's views.

"Herr Schiller," I began: *"Vicious, anti–Semitic, Nazi-lovers like you must suffer tremendous anguish and deep distress every time you read about the accomplishments of various Jews and the growing strength of Israel... While complete non-entities like you have no impact whatsoever on society, Jewish luminaries in science, art, politics, and academia grow brighter each year... Perhaps you can derive some joy in your vapid, vacuous life by standing nude in front of your bedroom mirror while you practice doing quenelles...."*

Gerald Schiller and, I'm sure, the ignominious Brian O'Neill and his cohorts at the *Post-Gazette*, thought that this letter had hit a new low, and that I had gone stark-raving mad. Hardly. But I do regret some of the expletives I used in my letter, which have been deleted here to maintain a "PG" rating. And my use of the word "quenelles" at the conclusion might require explanation for some. "Quenelle" is a word that originally referred to a French noodle or dumpling dish containing a mixture of creamed fish or meat. However, during and after World War II, it came to describe an obscene anti–Semitic hand gesture favored by French Nazis and other Jew-haters.

> TONY NORMAN: *Cyril has been abrasive with enough people and, in a way, that's just playfulness interpreted as hostility. He can be abrasive with me, but I know where he's coming from.*

If you go back through the years and review every one of my conflagrations with the local media, from my run-ins with DA Bob Duggan and Gene Coon, to this day, just look and you'll see who "lit the match." All I did was respond. But I've heard that, among local news people, unless you've received a letter of criticism from Cyril Wecht, you haven't really arrived professionally.

> WILLIAM ROBINSON: *Cyril is prolific in his writing and I think many of his letters have some historical value. Those of us who have received them probably have read them and chuckled a little bit. But I suspect that many of us did not take them as seriously as we should have.*

> TONY NORMAN: *Cyril is a two-fisted guy. He's a brawler. And he's sharp. But I think his need to be bare-knuckled, his loquaciousness and willingness to be "more articulate than thou" are also signs of a certain insecurity. He's big on his credentials. He's a lawyer and a doctor. He's this and he's that. He will tell you everything he's been and done. We get it. But at the same time, his aggression does mask some of his incredible accomplishments.*

In an effort to keep from being too bitter about my treatment in the local press, I always remind myself that, during my second courtroom drama, with the federal government this time, things reached a point at which the *Tribune-Review* and the *Post-Gazette* both ran editorials saying, in essence, "Put an end to this." They came around, and I certainly appreciated it.

So, have I ever experienced poor treatment similar to that which I encountered from the *Pittsburgh Press* and *Post-Gazette* from anyone in the local electronic media? The answer is "Yes." On KDKA radio, a man named John Cigna had always been friendly with me. I'd been on his program many times, and he liked to talk about JFK. But the day I was indicted in 1979, he turned on me. Cigna never called to see how I was doing and, I guess, just decided to go with the flow of the negative press. And there was another radio host at KDKA named Roy Fox. He didn't stay here long, but he had a talk show that was rather popular for a while. Fox was an arrogant person, and he also reveled in attacking me. So, yes, I experienced hostility in the press and on radio, too.

On the other end of the spectrum, one of my favorite talk-radio hosts was "Long John" Nebel, who broadcasted from New York City. From the mid–1950s until his death in 1978, he was a hugely popular all-night syndicated radio host, with millions of listeners and a fanatically loyal following. His program started at midnight, was broadcast until 6 a.m., and was carried nationwide, five nights a week. Somehow, someone got me invited to be on his show.

John wouldn't hesitate to rip you apart if he didn't like you but, if he liked you, you were in for a great experience. Any time I was in New York, I was on his show, and it was wonderful. I'd get there a little bit before midnight and, about 2:30 a.m., the bags would arrive from the Carnegie Deli. I was a younger man then and really enjoyed it, all the sandwiches, cheesecake, and so on. Anyway, we'd go on-the-air and talk about whatever—for five hours. Usually, John would take the last hour for himself. He and his guests would just go back and forth. If John was comfortable with you, he might even leave the room for a while. He and I really hit it off, and I was always a big success on Long John's show. I was with him probably a couple dozen times over the years.

Locally, I did something similar with Doug Hoerth on KDKA radio. To this day, if former listeners run into me on the street, they will say how much they enjoyed those shows. Somebody once told me that some of the old programs are still out there, on YouTube. But like John McIntire today, Doug was just too much for Pittsburgh. He was not delicate enough for local tastes.

JOHN McINTIRE: *Even though he is among the elites in Pittsburgh, Cyril has a "common-man's" sensibility. I love that about him. Once, I did a TV show for "Comcast On Demand" called, "Douchebags: People We Can All Live Without," and he actually participated in it, and used the word "douchebag" freely. I think I helped to win his heart by relentlessly rallying against the evil Mary Beth Buchanan, who brought that ugly, 84-count federal indictment against him. The only small tiff I had with Cyril was when he canceled an appearance on my show at the last minute and my director, during the live "Night Talk" show, found him on "Geraldo," at the same time. So, we put him up live on the air and made fun of him. I think he thought that was dirty pool. But I didn't want to blow my relationship with him, so we made up. Most people don't know that he's really sweet and has a great sense of humor. But if you piss him off, you'll find out the opposite side of Cyril, and it's not always pleasant.*

BEV SMITH: *When I was with the "American Radio Network" on WAMO, I did a series of four town hall meetings on the state of black Americans. They were held in Pittsburgh and broadcast nationally, and I brought people in from all corners of the country. I also invited Minister Louis Farrakhan, which became a major thing. A group of Jewish people contacted my management to make me uninvite him, and I resented them telling me who I can talk to about the black community. Farrakhan had done a lot in Chicago. He met with a rabbi and a Catholic priest every week and they formed a coalition. I don't agree with everything he says, but I respect him, and I wanted to hear his opinion about young black men and what could be done to help them.*

Some people told me that, if I sat on stage with Minister Farrakhan, I would lose my funding, and they were right. But Cyril Wecht read about it in the newspaper and sent a letter to me to tell me how proud he was of me—my mother has that letter—for sticking to what I believed. He felt that all voices had a right to be heard and that he and his wife wanted me to know that they think I'm a strong person. He didn't have to do that. I like him because he is who he is. He doesn't try to be anyone else. For him to send me a letter like that to me was so empowering.

Personally, I think that many of the ideas expressed by Minister Farrakhan are beyond the pale. To me, he's a charlatan, and a bigot. But I felt that Bev needed some support, so I offered it. I know what it's like to be in the eye of the storm when it comes to public and media pressure.

As for my career on local TV, I don't recall anything really negative happening to me. In fact, some TV people came to be quite friendly with me over the years. Adam Lynch (who I knew from the Pitt Players) and Eleanor Feeney both treated me well and fairly, and became close, personal friends. Nationally, the same is true, for the most part. The number of appearances that I have made on network and cable TV shows through the decades is significant. TV is the biggest "soapbox." Why not hop up there?

Collectively, I'm sure that I've appeared hundreds of times on television to talk about Elvis Presley, O.J. Simpson, Laci Peterson or Natalee Holloway; whatever cases were in the news. For a while, I was almost living at Videotech, in downtown Pittsburgh, with my friend Lou Cordera. Videotech maintains a TV set and the necessary satellite hook-up to project me from Pittsburgh to wherever, whenever I'm needed. I would go from one interview to another—three, four or five in a day, sometimes.

JIM RODDEY: *Television stations love Cyril. They know that, any time they need someone to talk, they can reach out to him. And he's so multi-faceted that he can talk on many subjects—government, law, medicine; whatever. They'll have Cyril because he is such a good interview.*

In this country, we have what everyone knows is "freedom of the press," but I will say this: I think the media onslaught is just too much these days. It has reached the point of supersaturation and redundancy that is, for me, unpleasant. Although I have appeared on countless TV programs through the years, I'll tell you what I hate about them: the extreme bias of some of the hosts, with Nancy Grace as the primary example. Her vicious attacks on people are not only disgraceful, but harmful, too. Remember, she was sued because one of her attacks allegedly drove a woman to suicide.

I met Nancy Grace early on, before anybody else even knew who she was. *Court TV* had launched a national show featuring Johnnie Cochran. Johnny filled the suit of "the black, male liberal." So, what was necessary, from the producer's viewpoint, to balance that out and create the "total TV package?" How about a white, conservative female—from the South, no less. So, *Court TV* created the beast.

I was never comfortable with Nancy because of her prosecutorial zeal. She snarls; there's no better word for it. Who covered the Casey Anthony case more than anyone else, perhaps, collectively? Nancy Grace. And I wasn't booked on her show at the time because I let her know what I thought of her. I cannot stand her and she knows it. So, she stopped calling. Good riddance.

The other thing I deplore about some of these TV shows is that many of the hosts, including some of whom I like and with whom I have appeared, adopt the attitude that "the more people we can get to talk about any subject at one time, the better." I'm not saying that it has to be me but, if I'm on, do you need another forensic scientist? If you have one defense attorney, do you need two? Do you need four or six people talking about the same topic at the same time? You've seen the "split-screen" set-up. It's like the old TV game show, *Hollywood Squares*. I won't do those anymore. I have learned that, if I'm not physically present, my microphone can be cut off at will, and I will be muzzled. Furthermore, I'm not going to lower myself to jumping into a screaming match with a bunch of pinheads. I abhor that set-up, and I've let it be known. I've said to producers, "I'm not telling you how to do your job or how to choose your guests, but if you call on me and intend to fit me in for only one or two minutes, along with five or six other people, I'd rather not be on your program."

In essence, my whole TV career began in 1968 when I did a program with Dan Rather about the assassination of JFK. What an arrogant S.O.B. Rather was—a prisoner of the media establishment who was, no doubt, on the rise and wanted to please his bosses more than he wanted to get to the truth. Dan Rather couldn't hold a candle to Geraldo Rivera, who is a smart and gracious man bent on exposing some of the ugly truths about our country.

In 1975, several years after the bombshell story was published, for which I was the source, in *The New York Times* about the President's missing brain, I was in Colorado skiing with my family during the kids' spring break when I got a call from Geraldo, whom I had never met, asking me to appear on his program about the JFK assassination. Of course, I accepted.

I started by driving my rental vehicle from Vail, with the Denver airport as my destination. And this was before they built the tunnel through Loveland Pass. Back then, you had to go up through a high pass in the mountains. Unfortunately, I couldn't make it through with the car and got stuck. I pulled over and, luckily, a trucker came by and gave me a lift. I just left the car there.

So, I flew to New York, did the program, and Geraldo took me to dinner afterwards at a French restaurant. It was the first time I had ever eaten "sweetbreads" (organ meat made from the thymus gland and pancreas of certain animals). I found them tasty, with all those wonderful herbs. Anyway, I made the round-trip in 36 hours, including a late-night flight from New York to Denver, and finished the ski trip with my wife and kids.

GERALDO RIVERA: *Cyril's expertise in terms of the [Kennedy] autopsy was invaluable. He was already well known back then as the go-to guy for commentary on forensic science issues.*

That was the beginning of my relationship with Geraldo, and I appeared many times on his various programs over the years. One time, I got a call from Jonathan Silver at the *Pittsburgh Post-Gazette* asking me how many times I had been on with Geraldo. I said, "I don't keep track." Apparently, they had made bets at the paper among themselves as to how many times I'd been on. Geraldo was still at ABC for that first show. And our relationship has been ongoing and friendly for 40-plus years now.

Geraldo Rivera is a law school graduate, and I find him knowledgeable and fair. He can be a little provocative and probing sometimes, but that's all part of the game. He doesn't let people get away with anything. I'm not sure what he believes about the

Warren Commission Report. I think he has a lot of doubts. But he has always allowed me to express my thoughts completely. Unfortunately, because of his latter relationship with Fox TV, he bent over backwards with that right-wing asshole, Bill O'Reilly, who "writes" books with titles such as *Killing Lincoln, Killing Jesus, Killing Reagan* and *Killing Kennedy*. (No, he hasn't written *Killing Wecht* yet.) I once appeared on that abomination called *The O'Reilly Factor*, and did not like the man.

Then one time, "Bill-O" appeared on Geraldo's show in a segment just before me to promote *Killing Kennedy*, but didn't stick around to debate me on the topic. He made his comments and left. Geraldo, however, was, as always, intelligent, articulate and interesting. I'm pleased to have had a relationship with him and am grateful to him for inviting me on all those programs. Once, when I had shingles, I appeared on Geraldo's show wearing an eye patch. When he signed off, he said, "Goodnight, Moshe Dayan." I'll never forget that.

Here's one last Geraldo story for you. A man named Larry Pozner, a lawyer from Colorado, was on the show with me to talk about the JonBenét Ramsey case. (Larry Pozner should not be confused with Gerald Posner, the author of *Case Closed: Lee Harvey Oswald and the Assassination of JFK*, who spent a couple of days in Pittsburgh interviewing me for that book.) Anyway, Pozner was a very arrogant guy, and we had some differences of opinion. At one point, I asked him if he had any experience in forensic pathology or forensic science. He had none, so I said, "I was doing medical-legal autopsies and working as a forensic pathologist when you were in short pants studying for your Bar Mitzvah." Well, Geraldo's crew just cracked up. And this was on live TV!

I've appeared on Geraldo's show and a host of others many times because of my involvement in high-profile crimes. Somewhere along the line, Larry King called. Over the years, I did at least a couple dozen Larry King programs. On one in particular, we were getting set to talk, for the "umpteenth" time about little JonBenét Ramsey. Around that time, the body of a young woman had been discovered in San Francisco Bay. She was from an Hispanic family, and nobody ever heard about her case. Do you think that if JonBenét Ramsey had been a girl of color she would have received as much attention as she did? Not on your life. She was a young, white, beauty queen from a rich family. During a break, I commented, "A pretty, blonde, white girl is killed and it becomes a national crisis. I see the bodies of poor brown and black children in the morgue all the time. Who will do shows about them?"

Another time with Larry King, I appeared alongside a forensic pathologist during Hurricane Katrina who actually said something to the effect of, "Never mind the dead bodies floating around in the water. It's not really a health problem." He didn't think people should be concerned about communicable, infectious diseases that will inevitably arise as the result of mixing sewage, human waste and decomposing corpses. So, I asked him, incredulously, "Where did you get your medical degree, sir? From Voodoo U.?" Immediately thereafter, Larry cut to a commercial. (I actually traveled to New Orleans at my own expense to help out after the Hurricane Katrina disaster. Over a three-day period, I conducted 30 autopsies for no charge.)

But my experience on national TV was not limited to Geraldo and Larry King. I appeared on all the programs. Name one. I was on it. Once, I did a show with Montel Williams, and it was a good experience. We had a discussion about racial issues. During the Iraq war, he had purchased one of the first Humvees, or "Hummers," which had become a big thing then. One day, Montel was driving in Manhattan and was pulled over by police. Why? I suppose it was because he was a black man driving an expensive vehicle. Luckily for him, the police didn't go "ape shit" on him, maybe because he was rich and famous. Two minutes later, they were asking for his autograph and tickets to his show. And while I did appear with Charlie Rose, unfortunately, I never did Phil Donahue. But I appeared with Maury Povich, for whatever that's worth. And I did *Dr. Phil* a couple of times concerning the Rebecca Zahau case, and he has said some nice things about me.

Local TV stations from elsewhere have contacted me, too. I made an appearance via Skype in San Diego about the suicide of Junior Seau, the football player. And I've done several international programs, especially on the Kennedy assassination, but on some other matters, too. One year, on JFK alone, I appeared on programs in Australia, England, South Africa and France, again, with the help of Pittsburgh's Videotech. I even got invited to appear on a program about JFK on *Al Jazeera*. The host came on and was unbelievably hostile. After two or three questions, I took my headset off, told him to go fuck himself, and left.

Surprisingly, *Al Jazeera* contacted me again some years later. At that time, the subject was "secret," although I deduced what it was. Yasser Arafat's body was about to be exhumed and they wanted me to consult with them about allegations that he had been poisoned with polonium by the Israelis. I was contacted to do the exhumation autopsy and had readily agreed. They called, we talked, but I didn't hear back. They must have checked me out and found out that not only am I Jewish, but I've made more than a few comments about Arafat and the Palestinians through the years. Not surprisingly, no future invitations came forth from them.

It's true that many of my most prominent media appearances have come about because of my connection to the JFK assassination case. If anybody calls, writes, or emails me for a consultation about that, I never ask, "How did you get my name?" or "Who referred you?" We can reasonably infer, considering my background and history, that my involvement with the subject is common knowledge to most members of the press. JFK provided me entrée into the world of the media, and my medical-legal perspective on cases of a high-profile nature was built on that foundation. At one time, I might have been seen as a bright, young guy with medical and law degrees who was willing to speak out. Now I'm older, but I still have some thoughts to share.

SANJAY GUPTA: *I met Cyril Wecht years ago when I was taking a course in forensics and he was one of the instructors. It was interesting to see how he approaches medical unknowns and medical mysteries. He is someone I often call when I'm doing something for TV. He's been practicing for a long time and is on the frontline as a pathologist. When I was doing a documentary for HBO called "One Nation Under Stress," I called him to get his take on some numbers and statistics we were reviewing. Did they make sense? After our conversation, Cyril spent a substantial amount of time on the phone with some from our team who had additional questions, and soon we realized that he'd be the perfect person to help us explain the facts about stress. So, we interviewed him, and he appeared in the documentary.*

I know what you're thinking. I must know a lot about stress because of the frenetic life I lead and my history of becoming outraged about many things at many times. Nothing could be further from the truth. I work hard, vent when I must, go on with my day, and sleep well at night.

SANJAY GUPTA: *There are people who are very busy, like Cyril, but they're not really stressed. And there are people who are not all that busy, and yet they're very stressed. The two don't correlate as well as people might think. I believe that Cyril is a good example of that. I'm trying to think if I ever saw him stressed when I've worked with him, and I can't say that I ever have.*

As much as I liked being a guest on the TV programs of others, I have to admit that having my own show was always an interest as well. But pitching TV programs is a crap-shoot. Even if you possess the greatest TV show idea ever devised, most of the time you end up with nothing. Henry Winkler, who played "Fonzie" on the hit sitcom *Happy Days*, once approached me about his interest in producing a TV series based on my casework. This was before *Forensic Files* appeared on cable, before Michael Baden's program, and before Henry Lee's program, too. Winkler had a great opportunity in his hands at the right time, but he turned out to be an asshole, and never got back to me. He screwed himself and me. He was just another Hollywood person.

Many years later, I got another opportunity to have my own TV show through a

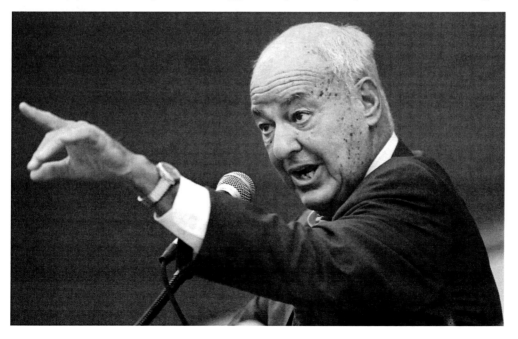

Making a point in the inimitable Wecht fashion (*Pittsburgh Post-Gazette*).

young man named Donnie Eichar, who had co-written and co-produced, among other programs, *Soaked in Bleach*, a film about the controversial death of rock start Kurt Cobain.

DONNIE EICHAR: *I pitched a TV series featuring Dr. Wecht in which he was to re-examine some of his most intriguing death cases. He and the people he worked with on them would review the cases, which would be presented as "mysteries." Dr. Wecht would then come in and solve them. The shows were designed as one-hour documentaries in which Dr. Wecht discovers new information, either as a consultant or as the forensic pathologist who did the autopsy, that would change the course of the cases. He would give his perspective, which might be different from what was presented in the media. The criteria that the network set is that Dr. Wecht's discovery had to "officially" lead to the case changing course, which narrowed down the case list.*

We shot a pilot called *The Body Detective*, which aired in 2016 on the LMN network. But as is all too often the case, the show was not picked up for a series. Another TV opportunity for me had bitten the dust, but it wasn't for lack of talent or effort on Donnie's part. Chalk it up to competition and the capricious nature of the television business.

On August 20, 2019, I traveled to Los Angeles to be interviewed by Oliver Stone for a new documentary he was producing about the JFK assassination. The interview lasted about two hours and I thoroughly enjoyed myself. While I've seen and have spoken with Oliver any number of times since 1990, when I consulted on his film *JFK*, it was a pleasure to revisit this important story in which we both share a great interest, complex as it is. He must have liked the performance and information he obtained from me in that interview because this email was waiting for me when I got back to my office the following day: *"Cyril, You were on top of your game. Never seen you so concise and strong. You truly are one of the Wonders of the World. I mean it. With Admiration, Oliver"*

MICHAEL BADEN: *I think Cyril is terrific. He is very good on the air. Many medical examiners talk in terms that the public can't understand, but Cyril doesn't do that. What I learned from him is that you must talk so that every person understands what you're saying. You must simplify things when you're describing. That's what makes him a good witness, and good on television.*

TONY NORMAN: *Say what you want about him, but Cyril's been a useful citizen. I think he's been an outstanding public servant. People say to me all the time, "You make fun of everyone, but you never make fun of Cyril Wecht." That's because I appreciate what he's done. I don't have the dislike of him that so many others do.*

ELLIS CANNON: *Cyril Wecht is among the most engaging, knowledgeable and well-informed guests I've had the privilege of interviewing. I have learned something each time, whether I was familiar with the topic or not. One of his most appealing qualities is his ability to discuss the complex and convey it in a means both colorful and informative, but also understandable. Dr. Wecht's vocabulary and encyclopedic recall of any number of facts, circumstances and evidence, in addition to his having the confidence to express opinions, many times on cases of great public interest, is what drew me and so many others to him. If he said something, he was to be believed. As he once reminded me, on-air:*

"It's OK to disagree, Ellis. We're friends." He encouraged me to offer contrasting points of view, which was extremely meaningful to me.

Bev Smith: *Generally speaking, when people get into their eighties, their passion dies. But Cyril's passion has not. He is the same as he always was. The thing that I admire most about him is that he is a man who does not compromise. I always introduced him on my radio show as a "truth-seeker" because that's what he is. He goes after the truth. And once he finds it, he will hold onto it like a pit bull. He will not let it go. We need more "Cyril Wechts" in this world.*

Tony Norman: *Cyril and I were having lunch downtown one day and, from the moment we sat down, a line of people began to assemble to speak with him. People came to our table to tell him how great he was. They made it clear that they believed in him, that he was "their guy."*

Federal Trial Part III
The Aftermath

In the wake of my federal corruption trial, reports from the jurors proved enlightening and all too telling about the methods and jurisprudence of Judge Arthur Schwab. Throughout the trial, he had "laid it on thick" with the jury. Schwab must have taken them for fools if he thought his tactics were going to get him what he wanted. He had cakes and cookies brought in to them regularly, which was very unusual and improper. In fact, it struck some of the jurors as "bizarre."

Schwab also brought in his cell phone to show the jurors pictures of his grandchildren. And when he took them into his chambers, another highly irregular move, he regaled them with explanations of his wall ornamentations. They weren't paintings but, rather, things that his wife had sewn—quilts, or something. He was trying to show them what a great guy he was, and at least five jurors didn't buy it. Judge Schwab tailored everything to try to convict me, and his jury charges were designed to direct them to do so. Why else would he curry such favor with the jury?

JERRY McDEVITT: *After the trial, I was so angry. I remember being on the courthouse steps when Schwab made the mistrial declaration, and I was asked what I thought. I said, "To be honest with you, I think a man should be entitled to a judge who reads the Constitution instead of cake and cookie recipes." Most lawyers don't talk about federal judges that way, but I had made up my mind that the Wecht trial was so ridiculous that I had to say something.*

DANIEL WECHT: *My dad came from an era in which people believed that justice would prevail in the end and, therefore, he always had a strong conviction that, when it came to his federal trial, ultimately, he would win. And he did.*

For the trial, Jerry McDevitt was the lead attorney, the hard-riding cowboy with a spine of steel. Mark Rush was an excellent "number two." I can't say enough about both of them. They worked tirelessly, all day and through evenings, and on weekends and holidays. The pace and workload of the case was murderous. And let me say here that Jerry's and Mark's junior K&L colleagues, paralegals and secretaries, were wonderful. They all were hard-working, dedicated and effective.

JERRY JOHNSON: *I represented Cyril in the beginning of his federal case, and left on good terms. I thought that he needed a bigger law firm, frankly, and he certainly got that with K&L Gates. What was most key in Cyril's defense, in my opinion, was Eileen Young. Her testimony went a long way toward winning the case. Cyril's lawyers, Jerry McDevitt and Mark Rush, were a very effective team, and they defended Cyril aggressively. The jury couldn't reach a verdict and, as any lawyer knows, no verdict means no conviction.*

Any number of people told me that Eileen was the key. She was the one who could talk credibly about what work I did for the Coroner's Office, what work I did for my private firm, and when.

ALAN JERRY JOHNSON: *When I was a U.S. Attorney, we'd consider, "Is what we're looking at a federal crime? And is it a crime that we can prove if we decide to prosecute?" After considering those two things, the third consideration was, "Is this worthy of prosecution at the federal level? Why would we get involved in this kind of case?" U.S. Attorneys represent the federal government, and are tasked with, in my opinion, handling big white-collar cases and big public corruption cases. We must be selective. The more cases we bring into the federal system, the harder it will be to take the time to prosecute those that we should be prosecuting, of which there are plenty.*

DAVID WECHT: *The whole federal case was a sham. It was vendetta-driven and an example of abuse of power and misuse of the prosecutor's office. It was also an example of abuse of power by law enforcement authorities. The U.S. Attorney's Office is not beyond reproach, nor is the FBI. They must always be scrutinized. In my dad's case, unethical prosecutors in league with unethical law enforcement agents attempted to drum-up as many charges as possible in the hope that they could get a conviction on at least one of them. That was their* modus operandi.

BOB BIBLE (JUROR): *As soon as the case was over, I thought that the prosecutors would have, at least, asked us what the vote was for each count. But without knowing, U.S. Attorney Stephen Stallings jumped up and said, "We're retrying." I'm thinking, "How much money did we already cost the taxpayers?" Without even finding out if the vote counts were close, they decided to spend more, which was very disappointing.*

JERRY JOHNSON: *It was shocking. Mary Beth Buchanan and her team had every opportunity as prosecutors to do what they could do, and failed. If I had lost that case, I'd have walked out and said, "The jury has spoken. We tried the best case we could, and the jury didn't find the defendant 'guilty beyond a reasonable doubt.'" But the prosecution immediately said that they intended to retry the case. When I heard that, I thought, "Wait a second. You better evaluate what you've done. You better see where the holes are because your case was shot up in a gunfight and, in the end, looked like Swiss cheese."*

After Arthur Schwab's mistrial declaration, we had, by then, given up on the Third Circuit throwing him off the case. My lawyers tried twice to do it. The first time, by a 2-to-1 vote, the Court left him in place. Just before the trial began, we moved again, and they swatted it aside.

JERRY McDEVITT: *I told the Court, "If you don't remove this guy, he will produce the biggest charade in Pittsburgh legal history," and he did. After the mistrial declaration, it was time to go back to the Third Circuit and I thought, "I'm going for double jeopardy; I'm not even going to mention Schwab again" because, if I did, it might appear as if we anticipated losing our argument. I had no faith that the Court would remove Schwab. If they had the appetite for it, they would have done it earlier. So, after filing our double jeopardy argument—18 pages about how Schwab had messed up the case—I received the Court's opinion. Unbelievably, in the last section, without even being asked, the Third Circuit removed Judge Schwab.*

First, the Third Circuit said that the interest of justice would be served by "fresh eyes on the case" and a "reduced level of rancor in the courtroom." Next, it found that Schwab had declared a mistrial "through a highly flawed set of procedures." It then cited cases holding that, even absent allegations of bias, the appearance of justice requires reassignment when a trial judge uses highly unusual procedures. The Court then concluded, "The problem today is not so much the appearance of bias as it is the appearance of litigation at a combative tenor that likely will not abate were Judge Schwab to remain on the case. We therefore direct that a less invested adjudicator take over from here."

JERRY MCDEVITT: *Rather than finding Judge Schwab to be a biased judge, they characterized him as an "invested adjudicator"!*

My case was then transferred to U.S. District Judge Sean J. McLaughlin of Erie, Pennsylvania. McLaughlin is everything you would want in a federal judge, which is everything that Schwab isn't. And make no mistake, the removal of Arthur Schwab made the difference for me. Think of all time and money that had been spent up to that point. All of it could have been avoided if Schwab had made the correct ruling in the first place by declaring the search warrants invalid. If he had, there would have been no trial. The government would not have spent millions of taxpayer dollars. I would have been able to preserve my nest egg to pass on to my children. And Jerry McDevitt would not have lost 31 pounds.

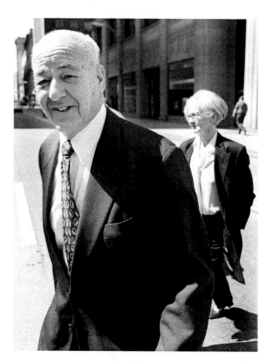

JERRY MCDEVITT: *The first thing that Judge McLaughlin asked us was, "Am I not bound by Judge Schwab's rulings on the law of the case?" I said, "No, and I'd like to brief you on that because there are case-dispositive issues here. If you agree with us, this case isn't going any further."*

By that point, I think the Third Circuit wanted the case aborted because they realized it was a bad prosecution and had become an embarrassment to the judiciary.

April 8, 2008. With Sigrid after a mistrial had been declared, effectively ending my federal corruption case (*Associated Press*).

JERRY McDEVITT: *We had two vigorous arguments before Judge McLaughlin, not on double jeopardy, but on whether or not he was bound, under the "law of the case doctrine," by Judge Schwab's rulings when it came to (1) his failure to dismiss substantive charges after the first trial, and (2) the validity of the search warrants.*

Unlike Schwab, Judge McLaughlin read all the briefs, which took about two months. Not long after we finished our second argument, he came out with his opinion. In his ruling, Judge McLaughlin did something that we thought was quite artful. By the time we got to him, the prosecution had dropped more of the charges they had filed against me. They were down to 14 from the original 84, some of which were just "666" charges (basically, for petty theft), which were total bullshit. By then, I had spent more than $4 million of my own money defending myself against an ever-shrinking list of counts, and I will go to my grave pissed off about that.

JERRY McDEVITT: *I presented our argument to Judge McLaughlin on those charges, too, to which he said, "I'm going to hold them in abeyance, but I am going to quash the search warrants. Ms. Buchanan can decide if she wants to appeal, and if she does and is successful, I'll come back and rule on these other arguments." I think the Judge was telling Mary Beth, "You can appeal, you might win, and we might have to come back here. But, if you do, I may just throw the case out on other grounds." It was his way of saying that there would be no second trial. And I'm confident he would have held to that because there were so many defects in the prosecution.*

MARK RUSH: *The motion that was granted by Judge McLaughlin was, in essence, the same motion we had made to Judge Schwab, only Schwab denied it.*

JERRY McDEVITT: *A year or so later, I saw Judge McLaughlin, walking down the street, and he said, "Jerry, I spent more time on those search warrants of yours than I've ever spent on anything." I said, "So did I. That's what offended me about Schwab. I put a lot of effort into trying to brief him on why those warrants were invalid, and he just wouldn't listen. You did."*

In short order, Mary Beth Buchanan dropped the remaining charges against me, in the most ungraceful and mean-spirited manner you can imagine, still vouching to the press for the validity of her failed prosecution. Buchanan had destroyed a lot of the credibility that our regional U.S. Attorney's Office had built up through the years. She totally disgraced the office. Unfortunately, Arthur Schwab will forever be a Judge, but he will never, I don't think, get promoted. His chances were destroyed by his handling of my case. He made a farce out of the whole thing, which I resent to this day. All citizens and taxpayers should resent this as well.

RICHARD THORNBURGH: *After the case was dismissed, I called for the Office of Professional Responsibility (OPR) to consider the same question that we asked from the very beginning: "Why was this case brought?" In my time as U.S. Attorney General, I fired U.S. Attorneys because they didn't hold to the standards that we wanted when filing prosecutions.*

MARK RUSH: *We filed a complaint against Mary Beth Buchanan with the OPR and the U.S. Department of Justice for her comments, because she said that Cyril was "guilty," but the jury didn't convict him.*

Soon after the case's dismissal, we held a news conference of our own, and I let it fly. I attacked Buchanan, rogue FBI agent Brad Orsini and, of course, Stephen A. Zappala, Jr., to whom I hurled out a challenge. I suggested that Zappala take a polygraph test to confirm whether or not he was the person who had been spreading the absurd rumor that I was seeking citizenship in Israel in case I was convicted. I also wanted Zappala to admit that he had said, "Anybody who fucks with me or my family is going to be indicted." I called-out "Stevie-Boy." Gutlessly, he never responded, and the local media never followed up, of course. It's always that way when it comes to Zappala. They're afraid of him because they know that he's willing to abuse his prosecutorial powers to settle scores. And, of course, they want access to his office in case a juicy trial comes along.

After the dismissal of my case, it was not as if I could simply go back to my work like nothing had happened. The new Allegheny County Executive, Rich Fitzgerald (a Democrat, mind you), made sure of it when he reneged on our agreement for him to reinstate me as Allegheny County's Chief Medical Examiner if I was cleared, in exchange for my support to help get him elected. Once in office, Fitzgerald made getting my job back a moot point by setting specific pretextual conditions for my employment, to which he had to know no one of my professional stature would agree. I would have had to clear everything that I said or did with some flunky in his office.

SOPHIE MASLOFF: *Even though I was angry with him many times, I had to admire Cyril because he has such courage. He could have pled "guilty" to one charge and walked away with probation, probably, but he wouldn't do it. Some of his friends advised him to do so, but he wanted to clear his name and get his job back. He fought hard but, in the end, he didn't get it.*

JERRY MCDEVITT: *Cyril's reputation and standing in the community can't be underestimated in a case like this. Our ability to bring out, through the prosecution's own witnesses, what kind of man he really is made the difference. But I have mixed feelings about him not getting his job back, because I believe that Zappala would have done it to him again. Cyril often says that the DA is a sociopath, and that's what worried me. If he went back to the Coroner's Office and did anything remotely questionable, he'd be prosecuted again. The "Zappala clan" has a history.*

EILEEN YOUNG: *I have a bad taste in my mouth because the whole case was a political vendetta, from day one. Dr. Wecht gave so much to Allegheny County. They had one of the most brilliant, educated and famous forensic pathologists in the world, and paid him a minuscule amount of money, yet he spent so much time in the Coroner's Office. He never worked "on the clock." He gave more than he ever received. People would call him on weekends and holidays, and he never said, "No." Allegheny County should have been grateful to have him.*

STANLEY ALBRIGHT (JUROR): *I'm of the opinion that you are what you think you are. This is where many people get messed up. They think poorly of themselves, so they think everybody else thinks poorly of them, too. Dr. Wecht doesn't think that way. He knows who and what he is.*

SAM SHAPIRO: *Most of my conversations with Cyril during those difficult times were over the phone, which is a little different than being right there in the room with him. But he never showed any weakness. He never showed any worry that he was going to be convicted. He always took the high road. We never once talked about what he was going to do if he went to jail. We always talked about those "no-good motherfuckers." Cyril is what he is and he never, ever is going to change his philosophy or his attitudes. He's a fighter. He's always going to win.*

In truth, I did consider, privately, what I would do if I was convicted and went to jail. I discussed things with Sigrid calmly, and talked about what would have to be done in our private office, from an economic standpoint. I'm not saying that I resigned myself to such a possibility, but I have always dealt with reality. I didn't know what was going to happen. Once it was over, of course, I was relieved.

MARK RUSH: *I used to walk down the street with Cyril during the trial and people would blow their car horns and wave. It was incredible. Jerry McDevitt and I were at the Capital Grille one evening having dinner. The TV news came on saying that the jury had hung, and everyone in the place started to applaud. It was clear that, in the battle of public relations, Cyril had won.*

JERRY MCDEVITT: *The media loves these trials. It gives them something to cover. The community probably gets a kick out of them, too. The Wecht case was entertainment for the whole city.*

ALAN JERRY JOHNSON: *Once the public got to see what the case was really about, they got sick of it. And I'm sure that any number of the jurors were thinking it even sooner, because they were sitting there and listening to it every day.*

DAVID WECHT: *The "presumption of innocence" goes out the window once the media spectacle begins. People tend to trust the government and assume that what the government says is correct. Many uninformed people go along with accusations that are made by government agents, so there's often actually a "presumption of guilt." The emotional and spiritual toll the trial took on my parents was enormous. They were not young, so the burdens were magnified. It was a difficult time for our entire family, but it was surely the most difficult for my parents.*

STANLEY ALBRIGHT (JUROR): *What happened in the Wecht trial is exactly what should have happened.*

DANIEL WECHT: *To my dad, the trial was just another challenge. He likes to think of himself as a kid who grew up in the Hill District, who was used to the rough-and-tumble. In The Hill, you don't back down from a fight; you don't roll over. That's a big part of who he is. How he was able to weather that trial, and weather it so well, may be one of his most amazing accomplishments.*

Strangely, what happened to me put me in a good position within the community. In fact, as part of his own political campaign, my son, David, conducted a survey to see where I stood with the public in the aftermath of my trial. In the Pittsburgh TV market, I had 83 percent name recognition and, if I recall correctly, a 56 percent approval rating, with only 12 percent disapproving.

For decades, I had been speaking out, in letters to the editors of our daily newspapers and on TV, arguing for things such as the legalization of marijuana, preserving a woman's "right to choose," analyzing controversial murder cases (including those involving police), repudiating anti–Semitism; you name it. How many people who are involved in such matters can boast of 56 percent approval? My trial, in some ways, propelled me back into the media and, after the fact, I was determined not to just walk off into the sunset.

JOE MANCUSO: *Actually, the publicity from the trial increased Cyril's business. When I first started with him in 1976 or 1977, we used to do autopsies on my lunch hour, or after work at my other job. We were doing 35–40 cases a year. In the years after the trial, we were doing 400–500. That was a considerable number for just two people.*

I knew that it would take me years to dig out from under my legal bills. As I've said, my federal mess cost me more than $4 million, and I didn't have that kind of money, so I had to borrow. (K&L Gates deserves great credit and my heartfelt gratitude for walking away from another $6.5 million that remained on their books.) I remortgaged our house in Squirrel Hill, and our place in Florida. I had maintained a solid investment portfolio, after 50-plus years of hard work, but had just a fraction of that left, which is nothing, given who I am and what I've accomplished. Sigrid and I couldn't live on what we had. Just take a look at what old-age homes cost these days. So, I was in no position to retire and, even today, I have no plans to do so. I can't afford to. When you take on the Feds, even if you win, you lose.

BOB BIBLE (JUROR): *I knew it cost Dr. Wecht a lot of money, never knowing the exact figure. But I know that Jerry McDevitt and the rest of the attorneys said that if they had to retry the case, they were going to do it for nothing. So, I figured he paid a "king's ransom" the first time. Before the trial started, obviously, I knew who Dr. Wecht was, but didn't know whether he was a good man or a bad one. My opinion going in was "whatever the facts tell me, that's what my opinion is going to be." As things went on, it became obvious that it was a political stunt for Mary Beth Buchanan. What a travesty that the government was willing to spend such a large amount of money on something as flimsy as this case was. Maybe they thought that, if nothing else, they could cripple Dr. Wecht financially, but I don't really know.*

BEN WECHT: *The trial was tremendously burdensome to my parents and would have crippled anybody but them. They are very strong. Getting up every morning and walking through a media gauntlet while being gawked at must have been awful. And reading about and hearing the ridicule and derision tossed around by people they once considered friends was hard for them.*

OLIVER STONE: *Cyril had to be a monster of energy to have overcome that. I asked him if the experience wore him down, because he still looked great. He said, "Well, I kept working every day." He thrives on work. Without it, he might shrivel up. Certainly, the accusations and loss of money was hard. And I knew he lost some friends, at least people he thought were friends.*

KERRY LEWIS: *Cyril was under indictment for a long time, and it was clear that the charges were petty and political. But the guy is incredible. He has a great reservoir of en-*

ergy. Most people, when they are propelled into the criminal system and the process drags on, get worn down. It zaps their energy. People tire and surrender. For Cyril, the more they threw at him, the stronger he became. He believed in himself and his work, and remained that way, even after the trial.

JIM RODDEY: *I can tell you from experience, not that I ever went through anything like Cyril went through, but being raked through the newspapers and television with negative coverage is very difficult to handle. You develop a thickness of hide but, unless you learn to shake it off, it can crush you. Cyril has had more of that than anybody I know, yet he holds his head up and never looks back. I know it always hurts him inside a lot, but you'd never know it.*

People who know nothing about how federal prosecutions work often ask, "Couldn't you get reimbursed for what you spent, given that the government failed?" There are laws that establish, in theory, that opportunity. But from a realistic standpoint, to do so, you would wind up having to retry your case. You'd have to show, unequivocally, that persons "A," "B" and "C" sat down in a meeting and said, "We're going to get Wecht." Malevolence and prosecutorial misconduct, in and of themselves, do not constitute the basis for you to recover what you spent on your defense, no matter how bogus the case was. I could have tried this, maybe against the county, but no lawyer was going to take such a case on a contingency, and how was I supposed to pay for it?

I'm certain that you could count on the fingers of one hand successful reimbursement actions of this nature. While it makes common sense that, as the victor, I should not have lost so much, I never think in a "Pollyanna-like" fashion about anything. What makes all of this even more egregious is the reality that everything that takes place in court is immune from civil action and defamation. The only thing you can do is re-challenge the government. They're going to be there forever, with unlimited resources, because they're playing with other people's money. And if you think that they'll say "We made a mistake," forget it.

Enough ruminating. What gives me great pleasure is the fact that Mary Beth Buchanan was destroyed by her actions. The last I heard, she had been bouncing from job to job and is now working in some piddling position outside of Pennsylvania. She's not destitute because she "married money." But she was never going to win appointment to the federal court, when she, in her own mind, had one buttock sitting on the bench of the Third Circuit. Then she got her ass whipped in 2010 by a more than two-to-one margin in the Republican primary for the U.S. House of Representatives by a then-unknown Keith Rothfus. The race should have been a slam dunk for her. But her prosecution of me killed her chances, and I couldn't have been happier.

RICHARD THORNBURGH: *Mary Beth Buchanan may have thought she had a promising career, but that went down in flames due to her ineptitude.*

DAVID WECHT: *There aren't many lawyers in Pittsburgh who have not just the ability but the courage that Jerry McDevitt has. He needed courage to stand up to the federal government and to Judge Arthur Schwab. Stanley Preiser was courageous like that. He was the attorney who had handled my dad's previous trial, with Allegheny County. It's good that my father had the wisdom to select those two great lawyers to fight against the power of the government.*

Another thing people ask me when talking about my trial is, "How did you handle the stress?" I have no magic formula. But I will say that having a wonderful and patient wife, four great kids and their spouses, and a bunch of grandkids, helped me immeasurably. And fortunately, I still had many loyal friends who remained with me through the thick-and-thin of it. When faced with the number of charges that were leveled against me, you have three choices: You can put your hand in the air, plead "guilty," and go off into the wilderness; you can commit suicide; or you can pick yourself up and fight like hell. I chose number three. I wouldn't have done anything else.

INGRID WECHT: *My dad was able to intellectualize things. He was an active part of his legal team, which, I think, helped. I went to the opening and the closing of the trial, and maybe one or two other days, but I remember the last day as being especially intense. Jerry McDevitt's closing argument was amazing. At one point, when he was speaking, another of his lawyers was patting my dad on the back. I was sitting right behind them and thinking, "This is just too much." It was draining. And yes, a lot of money was spent, but I would say that it was worth it.*

DAVID WECHT: *During the trial, our family continued to get together at least once a week; all of us. On a subtle level, my dad may have been more serious at that time, but it was a very incremental distinction. For the most part, he remained his old self. Let me illustrate it this way: My dad has always taken an active interest in not just the major issues affecting all members of our family, but minor ones as well; things as seemingly trivial as where my kids were going to have their meal on a particular evening, or how we were going to handle the kids on a weekend in which my wife and I planned to be away. He wants to help and wants everybody to be happy, safe, and satisfied. I don't know how he was able to maintain that equanimity and selflessness, because the overwhelming majority of people would have been wrapped up in themselves and their ordeal. But my dad was as directed toward his family's interests as ever.*

HAROLD BALK: *I'm a lawyer and, because I worked downtown, I went to more of the trial than anyone else. The court was just across the street from my office. So, I watched the proceedings and realized that the person on whom the trial had the greatest effect was my mother-in-law [Sigrid].*

JUNE SCHULBERG: *My heart went out to Sigrid because, within herself, she doesn't have the resources that Cyril has. She was always there to make life complete for him. I can't imagine what it was like for her, but I'm sure it was terrible. When I heard, before the trial started, who the judge was going to be, I said to Cyril, "That's going to be trouble." I knew Arthur Schwab.*

SIGRID WECHT: *We were in a state of siege. We were girded for battle, so to speak, and just moved ahead. During the trial, we functioned very well, amazingly. I was busy working every day while Cyril was in court. After court, he came back to the office and worked, too. He even did autopsies in the afternoons and on weekends. After the trial, it was more of a post-traumatic situation. I definitely changed. I'm not the same person that I was before all of it started. I have little interest and very little tolerance for certain types of people. I don't trust everyone. Cyril has powerful opinions and is an amazingly clear thinker. A lesser man would have buckled under the stress. In the law, they talk about the "reasonable man." Cyril is that person. But I am not the "reasonable woman." Inside, I was panicked and scared, so I tried to isolate, to retreat inward to protect myself from all the brouhaha. But Cyril always was and still is a "mind over matter" type of guy. His ability to handle things always amazes me.*

FRANCIS SHINE: *I saw Cyril in his suit on TV with his wife, going to court. They were often holding hands. And I never saw, not one time, Sigrid walking behind him. She was always beside or in front of him. That's not for show; that's just their nature. It's an automatic kind of thing.*

JOHN RAGO: *Cyril and Sigrid are like newlyweds. He teases her. She laughs at him. But I worried when the government went after Cyril's kids, David and Ben, that it could be the breaking point for him because I know how he is when it comes to his children.*

HOP KENDRICK: *Most people are intimidated by the government. Before the trial started, I asked Cyril, "So, they want you to plead 'guilty' to just one count. That's a far cry from 84. Why don't you do it?" "I can't," he said. I asked "Why not?" "Because I'll lose my medical and law licenses. If that happens, they win." I hadn't thought about it in that context. Then, one day after the trial was over, Cyril said to me that he didn't have the slightest idea just how unscrupulous the federal government could be. I said, "What difference does it make? You won." He said, "But do you know how much it cost?" I said, "I don't care how much. Thank God you had it to pay." "But I wanted to leave it to my children." I said, "Your kids have done well. They can take care of themselves. They don't need your money." I didn't know his wife was within earshot, but she leaned in and said, "Tell him that again. I tell him every day."*

There certainly were people, including my attorneys, who let me know what the consequences might be of playing things out at trial. "We can do this; or we can do that. These are the things to consider." And they were good attorneys. At the outset, however, they didn't know fully about the influence political players can have on individuals in Pennsylvania, or how malevolent Steve Zappala could be. My initial group of lawyers were simply looking at 84 felony counts and thought, "Why don't you plead 'guilty' to one, and we'll get you probation; no jail time, and it's over." Pretty tempting. So, yes, there were people close to me (but no one in my family) who felt that way, and some voiced their opinions to me directly or indirectly. That wasn't surprising. But they weren't considering what the political climate was at that time.

Mary Beth Buchanan was riding high. In her mind, she was headed for a lifetime federal judgeship or a senior position in Washington, D.C. The fact that I chose to put everything on the line, deplete my savings, and endure tremendous pressures, means much more when you take into account what I had to lose if I was convicted of even one single thing. To preserve my reputation, I chose to do battle against powerful forces, and I beat them. I've never heard of anyone who faced 84 counts in federal court who walked away in the end without calling a single witness. That has to be some kind of record.

BOB BIBLE (JUROR): *The whole experience scared me because, I was thinking, "If they can do this to somebody like Dr. Wecht, a well-known, respected individual, they could crush a normal person like me. It shows you to what lengths some people will go. I don't want to say I was naïve, but I thought the government would do what's right. I found out that's not the case all the time. They wanted Dr. Wecht to plead to something so they could say, 'Look, we got him.'"*

JOHN RAGO: *I always had faith that he'd get through his ordeal, but I worried about his health because you can only compartmentalize so much, I think. But Cyril kept working. He took his nightly steams. He kept his routine. He and his family really suffered an ordeal and I'm sure that he would say today, "I'm just fine." But how are you ever fine after something like that?*

I'm under stress every day of my life, but it doesn't bother me. For example, today, I went to the office, reviewed a bunch of cases to extract information to present at the national conference of the American College of Legal Medicine in a week or so, talking about police-related deaths. I was interviewed and had my picture taken by the *Pittsburgh Tribune-Review*, for one reason or another. Then I had to order food from two different places for our post–Yom Kippur family dinner the next day, after which I drove to East Liberty to speak at a funeral, and was interviewed by cell phone in the car on a radio show broadcasting in Detroit. I then returned to the office to meet with Sigrid and our accountants and, finally, headed out to conduct two autopsies. That's a typical day for me. No big deal.

DAVID WECHT: *The irony is that, at many points in my dad's career, he could have gone elsewhere and advanced himself professionally, but he is intensely loyal to Pittsburgh. He loves the city and would never leave. And how was he repaid for his loyalty? Prosecutors and agents, who acted purportedly in the name of the people (and on the people's dime), prosecuted him. The other irony is that my dad didn't need the Coroner's job to advance himself financially. To the contrary, he could have made much more money without it. The opportunity cost of putting in time at the County Coroner's Office versus doing private work was huge. If he was focused on making money, as the government alleged, he could have done far better by having nothing to do with government service. He could have hung out a shingle and done his work all around the world.*

JOE DOMINICK: *Cyril's federal trial was a waste of taxpayers' money. It forced him out of a position for which he was eminently qualified, and in which he should have remained. It left me with very hard feelings. I spent two weeks on the witness stand in that case and the prosecution could not prove anything that they alleged. The idea of going after a person who used county tax dollars to fund his own personal business is one thing; but when you indict a person for using county office equipment, that's ridiculous. I don't know of anyone who doesn't use the copier, fax machine, or telephone at work, at least some of the time.*

JOHN McINTIRE: *The thought that the U.S. Attorney's Office, in this age of terrorists and all sorts of dangerous criminals, was putting its effort behind prosecuting a man for, allegedly, sending a few too many private faxes from his public office, or having a member of his public staff drive him to the airport in a county car in lieu of a limo, was ridiculous. I blogged about it mercilessly and Cyril's secretary would print-out my posts and give them to him. He would read them and call me with such fervor to say, "I really appreciate your blogging, John. Thank you so much."*

In October 2007, when Dick Thornburgh testified to the U.S. House of Representatives at a hearing before the Committee on the Judiciary about "Allegations of Selective Prosecution: The Erosion of Public Confidence in Our Federal Justice System," predictably, Republicans were annoyed and Democrats were outraged. It seemed that the men and women on Capitol Hill were none too happy that the investigation was focused on the operations of George W. Bush's Department of Justice. And my case was just a small piece of it.

RICHARD THORNBURGH: *I said, "I'll tell you the story and you can draw your own conclusion," and laid out the circumstantial evidence that indicated why Cyril's case had been brought. Did I know why? Not really. But I could "read the tea leaves," as they say, and knew what it looked like.*

ALAN JERRY JOHNSON: *I was shocked that such a thing [as firing U.S. Attorneys for not prosecuting particular types of people] could happen in the Department of Justice. They treated the attorneys like they were a bunch of political hacks that could be fired at will. Many of the attorneys they fired were among their best, and the reason they got fired is because they wouldn't follow the Party line. I felt for every one of them. When George W. Bush put Alberto Gonzales in the U.S. Attorney General's Office, everybody asked, "Where did he come from? What is his background?" He had none. Bush could have appointed somebody better than him.*

At the National Association of Medical Examiners, I was a member of a special committee called "The Independence of Medical Examiners." The chairwoman, Dr. Judy Melinek, a forensic pathologist from San Francisco, assembled the committee and introduced a resolution. Mine was the leading case within the resolution and details were shared about how the political system came down on me for my independent stance. My colleagues were shocked to hear how much money it cost me to defend myself, and the resolution was adopted, to my great satisfaction.

RABBI ALVIN BERKUN: *Cyril could have retired years ago, but that federal case took so much out of his well-being financially, and every other way. He works so hard. He travels all over giving expert testimony and doing autopsies. The number of cases that come his way regularly is amazing. Cyril is a proven master of his craft, and it's nice that his peers have recognized that.*

GERALDO RIVERA: *I want to say something about the jam Cyril got himself in. The federal case was, to me, unfair and, on its face, did not ring true. It certainly didn't jibe with the Cyril Wecht that I have known for decades now. I was confident that he was going to "beat the rap." I know that period in his life was a very tough time for him. I still put him on TV and never wavered in my support, not just because of his credibility as a scientist, but also his integrity as a person.*

DONALD GUTER: *I was there for the investigation, and felt so bad for him. Some people he knew just ran and hid. So, I wrote a piece [for a local newspaper] in his defense because I thought that no one should abandon a friend when that friend needs you.*

JOE DOMINICK: *Cyril was under a lot of pressure during the trial, but he handled it. The man is not able to be shaken, and that's what's amazing about him. He's at a different level than everyone else.*

MARK RUSH: *We knew that we could paint a picture of a man who truly dedicated every ounce, every fiber of his existence to forensic science. It was clear what Cyril had been doing for Allegheny County, and the surrounding counties.*

BOB BIBLE (JUROR): *The Wecht trial was the first time I ever got called for jury duty. I really didn't want to go, but I was glad I did it. It got to be pretty obvious toward the end that all Mary Beth Buchanan was trying to do was put a feather in her cap by frying Dr. Wecht and moving up to bigger and better things. I thought, "What a scam this is."*

BRUCE THOMAS (JUROR): *I remember one high-powered lawyer from Chicago. He seemed to detest being there, and wasn't a good witness for the prosecution. They asked him what Dr. Wecht's rate was and what he was allowed for expenses. He said, "We didn't care. We wanted him."*

I've often said how grateful I am for those who stuck with me. The district attorneys and coroners of the surrounding counties; not one of them dropped me. And there were some private attorneys who were just wonderful, too. A few of them told the federal government, "Go screw yourself," when they were called by phone to talk about the "Smith" case or the "Jones" case, and so on. Others, you can understand, got frightened or buckled under, but nobody turned on me. The prosecution was calling around with a goal: "Can we get anyone to say Wecht is an asshole?" No way. People spoke glowingly of me.

MARK GERAGOS: *That prosecution was such a travesty. I was actually listed as one of the "victims." I told the prosecutor, "This is ridiculous." Take a look at the indictment. You'll see "M.G." That's me. I said, "I'm not complaining. If anything, Cyril's charges were a bargain."*

SAMUEL HAZO: *Cyril is pretty outspoken; sometimes a little "over-spoken," about his convictions; but that's the man. You have to accept that if you know him. The case they brought against him was politically motivated. It was dripping with malice. How he survived, I'll never know.*

GARY AGUILAR: *You basically have to stick your fingers in their eyes. That's the way the game is played. I grew up on the streets of Hollywood, one of 12 kids. I can get down in the gutter and fight better than most, and Cyril has inspired me to not take injustice lying down. He is built on a bedrock of moral indignation and has a thirst for justice that drives his every move.*

KATHY MCCABE: *I don't know why it was so important for somebody to do that to him. He wasn't doing anything that anybody else wasn't doing. It was a waste of taxpayers' money. What they did was hurt him in the pocketbook. They didn't hurt his popularity because people still know him and still like him.*

MARK RUSH: *Here was a man who was fighting for his freedom, to save a lifetime of work, his reputation and his family. The federal government was throwing charge after charge at him yet, when I would call him to talk about the case, the first thing he would ask me was, "How are your children?" He still asks me that.*

JOHN PECK: *There are not many people who could have withstood and recovered from the two criminal cases that Cyril's had to defend. He simply took them in stride. I've had jurors tell me how impressed they were with him as an expert witness and, obviously, the jury for his federal trial was impressed with him as a defendant. They didn't care for the prosecution's case at all.*

ROBERT TANENBAUM: *It came with a great cost to Cyril, but his strength and character showed through. He's an extraordinary person; a great American. He's the kind of person I'm proud to call a friend. Cyril is the kind of guy who would have been at Guadalcanal charging forward.*

EILEEN YOUNG: *I wished that they would have acquitted him totally, because I felt that was the only fair thing to do. To tell you the truth, the worst thing that happened to me was losing my job, which was a very important part of my life. My attorney said that she would represent me, but I could not be working in the Coroner's Office. She said that it was not in my best interest. So, I retired, which was heartbreaking. Nothing could be as exciting as the job I had working for Dr. Wecht. It was different every day, and always interesting. I miss it to this day.*

BOB BIBLE (JUROR): *After the trial, the FBI called me and wanted to talk. I was worried because, given what they had tried to do to Dr. Wecht, and me being the foreman of the jury, I didn't know whether they were going to try to pin something on me.*

DAWN CASHMERE (JUROR): *The FBI started calling all of us jurors. I talked it over with my husband and said, "I'm not calling them back. I don't have to. This is a done deal." My husband said, "Fine. Just be aware that they could come and make our lives miserable if they want."*

For the FBI to call jurors after a case has been adjudicated, is unheard of, but they did it—no doubt at the behest or, at least, with the approval of that miscreant and scoundrel, Brad Orsini. It was rank intimidation. Most people never learn about this type of shady behavior that, at times, is undertaken by our agents of law enforcement. What were the jurors to do? If the government chose to retry me, the court would have empaneled a completely new set of unsuspecting citizens. The only reason for FBI agents to call them was as an act of retribution, to instill fear and paranoia, and to mess with the lives of the people who dealt them their loss in court.

BOB BIBLE (JUROR): *Two weeks after the trial, we agreed to get together with Dr. and Mrs. Wecht and their attorneys to have a meal and discuss the case. They said to us, "If there's going to be a retrial, we'd like to know how we did and what we could do better the next time around."*

BRUCE THOMAS (JUROR): *We wanted to give them tips about what impressed us, and what didn't play well; and what the sticking points were for the jurors who didn't believe them.*

DAWN CASHMERE (JUROR): *Dr. Wecht also tailgated with us at a Pittsburgh Pirates baseball game. People were coming over to say, "Hello" to him and shake his hand. That was very good to see.*

BOB BIBLE (JUROR): *One time, Dr. Wecht started telling us about some of his cases, and I was thinking, "I would love to be in a bar with him." I'd sit there and let him talk all night long.*

I Did It My Way

INGRID WECHT: *On one particularly beautiful day, my dad had no autopsies to do and, instead of relaxing and enjoying himself, he told me that he felt like the whole day was wasted. He said, "Baby, this is a good example of why I wouldn't want to retire. What am I going to do all day?"*

Most people my age aren't doing much anymore. They may have spent decades becoming physicians, attorneys, educators—what have you—only to say, "Now I'm 65, and I'm retiring." But I believe that, in 2020, retirement age should not be 65. It should be 75, 80, or even later. If one is in good health and able to do his or her job satisfactorily, what difference should it make?

One evening, at a political fundraiser for my son David, a man approached me and introduced himself. He was the son of a former medical-school classmate of mine, and a successful orthopedic surgeon in his own right. Naturally, I asked him, "So, what is your father doing these days?" and he replied, "My dad retired 20 years ago," to which I responded, "Is he OK?" "Oh, yeah," the man said. "He spends a lot of his time in New Castle (Pennsylvania) at his cattle farm."

Throughout my life, I've known people like this; people who have accumulated money enough to live comfortably, then just "pack it in." And there's nothing wrong with that. It's their right. But if one decides indeed to pack it in, shouldn't he or she then do something of a substantive nature? How about community service? Or, if one always wanted to be a writer or a painter, why not pursue those activities? But a cattle farm? Maybe my old classmate always wanted to be a cowboy. The way I see things, you have but one life to live, man. Do what makes you happy. And apart from my family, what makes me happy is my work. And I always work very hard, even now.

DAVID WECHT: *My dad is still working full-time at his profession, at age 89. He continues to do many autopsies every week, often multiple autopsies in a single day. He has unique energy, a unique drive, and incredible willpower. He's a remarkable man. There's no one like him.*

To be sure, the world is full of people who work hard. But there are very few who work with the intensity that I do, given the volume and overall variety of the demands placed on me and my time. On any given day, I'll receive letters from people who are in need of assistance, and calls from lawyers who represent people who may or may not have done questionable things. I might be asked to deliver a speech or a lecture, or draft a report on this case or that. I may also conduct an autopsy, all on top of dealing with a host of family and personal matters. I might fit in a little screaming and yelling, too. That's my nature. But because I have maintained high standards for myself and my own productivity, I have expected a lot from my colleagues and my family. For my kids, carrying the name "Wecht" has sometimes been a burden.

> DAVID WECHT: *I never felt that there was any undue pressure to excel or to go in any particular direction. On the contrary, we had a relaxed and delightful upbringing because our family has always been very close. My parents have always been loving, caring, involved, and generous to a fault. They seldom ever said, "No," to anything that my brothers, my sister, or I wanted.*

All four of my kids are graduates of Shady Side Academy, which is a private school, where they did well. Of my children, David is the oldest. He's a "double graduate" of Yale University, having received his B.A. from Yale College and his J.D. from Yale Law School. He is now a Justice of the Pennsylvania Supreme Court. He and his wife, Valerie, have four children.

Daniel, my second son, is a Harvard graduate and also earned a Harvard master's degree in anthropology. He then received his medical degree at the University of Pennsylvania, and is now a practicing neurosurgeon in Pittsburgh, at the University of Pittsburgh Medical Center (UPMC). With his wife, Anna, Danny has three kids.

My youngest son, Benjamin, is a graduate of the University of Pennsylvania, and earned a master's degree in writing from Stanford. He was formerly a reporter in Maine and Connecticut, but returned to Pittsburgh and worked in public relations for UPMC and Carnegie Mellon University. He is now program director of the Cyril H. Wecht Institute of Forensic Science and Law at Duquesne University. Ben and his wife, Flynne, have two children.

Finally, my daughter and youngest child, Ingrid, is a graduate of Dartmouth College. She then received

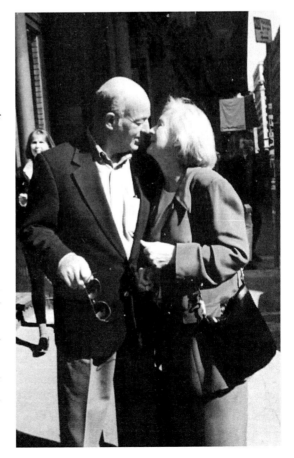

A tender moment with Sigrid.

both her master's and medical degrees from Georgetown, and did her residency in obstetrics and gynecology at West Penn Hospital in Pittsburgh. She's a partner here in an OBGYN group, is very active in her community, and is a wonderful mother. With her husband, Harold Balk, she has two kids.

Sigrid, my dear wife, as you've learned, grew up in Norway as a Lutheran, but converted to Judaism, as did David's and Danny's wives. Ben's wife was born Jewish and so was Ingrid's husband. None of us are Orthodox, nor are we very religiously observant, to be honest. But all of us are very proud Jews.

Once the kids had been raised, Sigrid went back to school and earned a master's degree at the Graduate School of Public and International Affairs (GSPIA) at the University of Pittsburgh. After that, she went on to get a law degree from Pitt. For several years, Sigrid and I operated our own law firm in partnership with our son, David, before he became a judge.

All my life I've been busy as hell and, sometimes, I get a little tired because my workload is very heavy. I always had two or three different jobs, and have been around the horn, speaking all over the place. I have given as many as five talks in a day; two or three per day has been quite common.

DAVID WECHT: *My dad invented multitasking before it had a name. He's incredibly busy and likes it that way. Even on vacation, he'll read files, call the office, speak on the phone with lawyers, and so forth. My dad loves his work more than anyone I've ever known.*

MICHAEL BADEN: *It's amazing how many cases Cyril does at his age, now. Most forensic pathologists retire in their 60s and go and play golf somewhere. I don't understand Cyril fully. It must be because he loves what he does. But, at the same time, I've spent time with him at his home, and he is a great father and husband. He always finds time for his family.*

When the kids reached high school, I made sure to be in the stands to watch their exploits on the athletic field, and I remember thinking about how few parents were present to cheer for their kids. I knew damned well that none were as busy as me, and thought, "Look at what they're missing." I'm very, very proud of my children, their beliefs and attitudes, their honesty, and their industriousness. Sigrid has had the greatest influence on them. (Mothers usually do.) She deserves most of the credit for the healthy and happy lives they lead.

SIGRID WECHT: *Our children were good kids. They were self-motivated. We didn't have to push them. Now that I have grandkids, I see how different each succeeding generation can be. These days, you have to watch kids more closely, and guide them much more than we ever did.*

As only children, it was important for both Sigrid and I to have a family, but we never decided to have "X" number of kids. If there had been three or five or six, that would have been fine. I don't know why we ended up with four. We just did. Anyway, I'm very happy about the fact that my kids all like each other. They invite each other to their homes when Sigrid and I are away. For me, family is my number one priority. If one has a good family life, everything else is gravy.

Of course, it's good to be healthy. It's nice to make a good living and to be professionally successful. And it's good to have friends by whom one is admired and respected. But there are people who have all of this and yet don't have a comfortable relationship with their spouses or an easy rapport with their children. Fortunately, I have these things, and I am grateful for them.

For Sigrid, life with me hasn't been easy. She has the "patience of Job," but she's no push-over. Sometimes she will "let me have it," without hesitation. But somehow, our relationship flows nicely. We have some disagreements, but no bitter quarrels. And we've developed a lifestyle of getting up together in the morning, and going to bed together at night. We both like movies and, to some extent, the same kinds. We enjoy the same friends, although most of them are mine because, being originally from Norway, Sigrid doesn't have any childhood friends who live locally. Sigrid has brought stability to the lives of myself and our children, and I am very proud—and very lucky—to have had her by my side. I've needed her more than she will ever know, especially during trying times.

STUART GRODD: *Sigrid must be an extraordinary woman to keep up with Cyril and that whole family. Cyril could never have done what he's done without her. She's a big, big part of his life.*

At 89, I still make a decent living, and I must because, remember, my federal case cost me more than $4 million, which is a big chunk of cash. What bothers me most about that is the fact that I would have liked to have left that money to my children

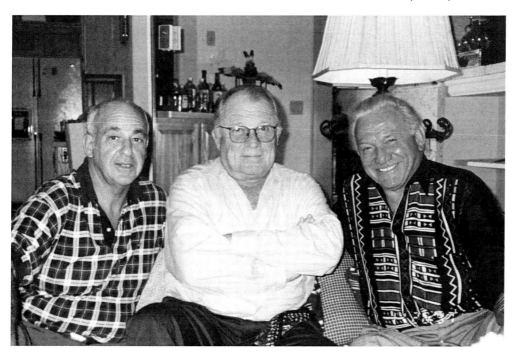

Me, legendary lawyer F. Lee Bailey, and Stanley Preiser. Stanley was the attorney who defended me in my first public corruption trial.

and grandchildren. Today, a high-quality college education costs about $70,000 per year for tuition, room and board, for starters. All my grandkids are bright, and their parents are sending them to fine schools, but I would have liked to have been able to foot the bill for them. That's what really, really hurts.

As a professional, lawyers know that they'll get from me candor, fairness and decency, whether it's in a deposition or on the witness stand. I'm proud of the fact that, even with my big mouth, and all the positions that I've taken throughout my career, I still maintain a large degree of acceptance, admiration and respect. But I'm not so sure that I have achieved everything that I could or should have in my life. If I had been a bit more diplomatic and patient, and a little less antagonistic and controversial, I might have achieved more. But it's idle speculation at this point.

> SIGRID WECHT: *I do think that Cyril has some anger about getting older. Physically, he has some aches and pains. And if he could learn to sit still for a while, he could spend his days reading and writing. But I'll tell you this: It's been an interesting ride being his wife. I have no regrets.*

> BEN WECHT: *People see a hard exterior by way of media portrayals of my dad and because of some of the fights he's been in, all of which he, generally, didn't start. But he's a total softie and extremely generous.*

> DANIEL WECHT: *He invites people to meals and picks up the tab. He offers rides to anyone who needs one. He gives things away. If somebody he knows is coming to town, he insists on hosting them in his home. And he not only wants to have his kids and grandkids over, but he welcomes their friends, too.*

> OLIVER STONE: *Cyril Wecht is a very admirable man; very straightforward and easy to talk with. We had a wonderful dinner together in Pittsburgh and I met some of his kids. His wife was lovely. It was a very warm meeting. He has a great family life, which was very inspiring to me.*

> JOSH SHAPIRO: *I found Cyril to be a person of serious substance with deeply held convictions and beliefs. We bonded over a number of things that had nothing to do with politics. We both think very seriously about family and faith. I talked with him about how to balance family life and politics, and how you weave your faith into that, and I enjoyed those conversations very much.*

> DAVID WECHT: *My dad is a genuinely open person with an incredibly hospitable spirit. And he's very trusting despite the hostility to which he's been subjected. As a former judge and now a Pennsylvania Supreme Court Justice, a lot of my electoral success is due to him. I have received many votes from people because they love and respect my dad. He has been a great asset to me in all of my campaigns. His love and advice have always guided me in the right direction.*

> HAROLD BALK: *If you really knew Cyril Wecht, you would love him.*

> BEV SMITH: *I keep wishing there was another Cyril Wecht so I could marry him. Every once in a while, you'll meet a really special person and, in this city, for me, that person is Cyril. He is in the "human-being business." I hope that I live to see the day when he will be properly recognized as a "favorite son" of Pittsburgh, because no one deserves it more than he does.*

Hop Kendrick: *Cyril has been entirely consistent in his beliefs throughout his whole life. He's always been willing to stand up, especially for the little guy. I've never met a man who is more honest, outspoken and committed to improving the quality of life for the community than Cyril.*

Dawna Kaufmann: *He is as concerned about justice for the family of a murdered child as he is for the victim of a racially motivated police shooting, and he won't stop until he finds out exactly what happened to the unfortunate individual resting on the slab in his morgue.*

Mark Geragos: *So much of his work is correcting injustices before they happen. It's truly astonishing. I think it's a tribute to the fact that he doesn't really come with any kind of an agenda, except for a healthy dose of skepticism. Most of law enforcement look at coroners as an adjunct. It's almost like they have a theory and they want the coroner to fit into it. That's one of the reasons that Cyril stands out. It's a blessing and a curse for him. It's a blessing in the sense that he does not allow himself to be co-opted by law enforcement and, at the same time, it's a curse because he makes enemies when he won't dance to their song.*

Katherine Ramsland: *People have strong reactions and responses to Cyril. He is a very controversial figure. He's controversial because he's outspoken, and his outspokenness has helped to make our field more accountable. Behind the scenes, he's been very much a part of the movement to make our field respectable. When we say that we're using science, we're using science. We're not just sloughing off, doing things superficially, and pretending that it's science. Some people don't like his outspoken ways, but that's what makes him who he is.*

Susan Shanaman: *I knew of Cyril Wecht for many years before I had ever met him. Primarily, I knew him as a pathologist who does many autopsies for the coroners in the western part of Pennsylvania. He is a very bright individual, and he's known for his competency. He is, obviously, well known and well recognized for the work that he does, nationwide. And that is not to say that he has not engendered some controversy here or there. But then again, my theory is, if you're doing your job, that comes with the territory.*

Donnie Eichar: *Dr. Wecht has a great command of the art of storytelling, but in a very informed, factual, science-backed manner. I think that's why he is so successful. He reminds me of a renegade cowboy who happens to be a forensic scientist, and he just doesn't give a damn what anybody thinks. He carries a big gun and he knows how to use it. The big gun is his intellect, his encyclopedic memory, and his knowledge of the law.*

Richard Sprague: *On a personal level, Cyril has a heart of gold. There's never been a time when I've asked him for something that he's not knocked himself out trying to be helpful.*

Jennifer Hammers: *I've learned from my experiences with Dr. Wecht that you can have a long, interesting, enjoyable, and successful career in forensic pathology, if you do it in a way that energizes and fulfills you. You have to be brave and not worry about what other people think.*

Tom Noguchi: *I'd do anything for Cyril. He is an amazing man. I juggle four or five projects at one time and sometimes can't do it. How many projects does Cyril juggle? Many more than me, I'm sure. He is like a magician, and he's been able to do that for a very long time. There is no person like Cyril Wecht, and I don't know if we're going to see anyone like him in the future.*

SOPHIE MASLOFF: *Cyril believes every word he says, from the bottom of his heart. He isn't in the game for the glory or the publicity. When you're in politics for as long as I was, you can develop a jaded outlook when it comes to politicians. Some of them couldn't earn a dime in any other line of work, anywhere. Cyril got involved in politics because he believed in things. That's what I have always admired about that man. There will never be another person like him.*

MARK RUSH: *The public only sees the Cyril Wecht that's on the news, using the big words or calling someone out. But in truth, he is incredibly caring. One time, my daughter was having headaches. She had no history of migraines, and her primary care physician couldn't figure out what was wrong. Who did I call? Cyril Wecht. First thing the next morning, my daughter was being examined by the head of neurology at Children's Hospital. Cyril just made a phone call.*

ROBERT TANENBAUM: *I have the utmost respect and love for Cyril. My feelings are based upon his expertise, honesty, and independence. He's the best example of "American exceptionalism."*

JOSIAH THOMPSON: *I have a theory about why Cyril's so healthy. He's a happy man. His energy is so high because he's happy with his life.*

FRANCO HARRIS: *I run into Cyril, from time-to-time, at events around town, and even sometimes at the airport. I have always had great respect for him, given his long track record as a warrior for social justice. Cyril's done a lot for Pittsburgh. And his efforts have served to fuel debate and discussion about many important cases and issues, both locally and nationally.*

KERRY LEWIS: *I like Cyril because of his spirit. You see someone like him and you say, "Now, that's a man. That's what real guts is."*

BOB DEL GRECO: *Cyril is passionate. Within the legal community, on many occasions, people believe that the outcome of a case could be determined by who gets to Cyril Wecht first. There can't be any higher praise than that. If there is an unexplainable death, oftentimes the first thing that anyone says is, "Call Cyril Wecht." If you have him, you'll have a leg to stand up on.*

ROBERT TANENBAUM: *Cyril Wecht is a classic "great American." He calls things as he honestly sees them. He's straightforward and is capable of explaining key points and making them very clear. And he can back things up with scientific data. I've always admired him. Integrity, intellect and independence; that's Cyril.*

GERALDO RIVERA: *Cyril is a no-nonsense, straight-talking expert. He's a renowned scientist who has little patience for rigmarole or politics. He gets right to the point and doesn't really care whose feelings get hurt. Cyril speaks to the forensic truth of what his investigations and examinations reveal.*

MICHAEL BADEN: *Cyril has been an important factor in my professional life. He really mentored me, in some ways. He was always encouraging. He brought me in to a senior position at the American Academy of Forensic Sciences and I have, from time to time, discussed cases with him. And even though, sometimes, we disagree, I think that he has good opinions. What Cyril does is raise important issues, and the most important is that the medical exam-*

iner has to be independent of what is beneficial for defendants, defense attorneys, prosecutors and plaintiffs.

ALAN DERSHOWITZ: *I think he was the first and best, and he's still the standard.*

Consider the world, the centuries and the generations. We're here for just a bit of time. In a way, it makes you feel like no more than a grain of sand on a vast beach. Who are we? What's this all about? You were born and you're going to die. This is your one shot, so make it a good one. I really don't believe in an afterlife. But I truly envy people who have strong beliefs in this regard because I think it would make life and getting old much easier.

DANIEL WECHT: *It's kind of a Jewish tradition. You make your mark in this life. When my dad thinks of the afterlife, he probably thinks about his parents, with whom he was very close. But I doubt that he gives much thought to what will happen once he's gone. He's not too inwardly reflective. He's very much in the present.*

As I grow older, I don't have a fear of death. What saddens me is the fact that, when my time comes, I will no longer be with my wife, children and grandchildren. But here's the other thing that bothers me: Almost all of my close, personal friends, whom I have loved and who have meant so much to me, have already gone, or will go soon. I'm bitter about that. But bitter against what?

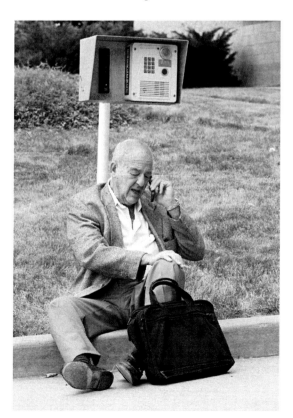

Business as usual, 2009 (*Associated Press*).

DANIEL WECHT: *I think, at some level, my dad thinks about his mortality. But his energy doesn't speak of desperation. He's not tired. He may live forever.*

JOSEPH MAROON: *Cyril, at 89 years old, is still a paragon of energy, cognitive awareness and articulateness. When it comes to his recall of facts and detail, he's as sharp as I remember him being thirty years ago. I don't know what anti-aging program he's on, but I want to be part of it.*

SUSAN SHANAMAN: *I hope that when I'm his age, I'm trucking along as well as he is. He still has "it," both in spirit and in his mind in terms of doing his job and doing the right thing.*

KEN GORMLEY: *I remember attending an event in the all-purpose room at St. Anselm in Swissvale, when I was in grade school, and hearing Dr. Wecht speak about the Kennedy assassination. That was more than fifty years ago. Fortunately, I've had the privilege to in-*

teract with Cyril throughout my career as a lawyer and legal educator. He's just as sharp, witty and captivating as he was 50 years ago.

I hope this book has answered some questions you may have had about me. Few people undertake a project such as this without a healthy ego but, while I am happy to tell my story, it's not egotism that drives me. My goal has been to explain, once and for all, what happened to me, and to let people know what my family, friends, acquaintances, and those who have followed my trials, came to know. I want them to understand what goes on behind the scenes in this country in terms of political misbehavior, police violence, and prosecutorial bias, and the kinds of reprehensible things that are done every day by those in power. I want people to understand that the FBI is not such an upstanding organization, one that would never do anything improper, unethical, immoral, or illegal. I want people to understand how court cases can be manipulated and how judicial misconduct can overrule facts and reason.

Many people think that when a judge dons a robe and raises a gavel, it leads to objectivity and a dispassionate approach to every case. That is very far from the truth. Appointed judges are probably more dangerous than elected ones because of their political ideology, and don't tell me that they don't have one. Think about it. A federal judge is appointed for life and then can do whatever he or she wants. I'm sure that very few federal judges in the 244-year history of our great nation have been removed from office for misconduct. Once they're in, baby, they're in.

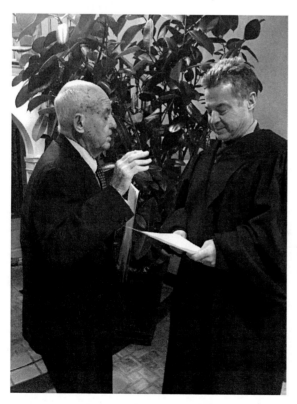

Being sworn in by my son David as a newly appointed member of the Pennsylvania Coroners' Education Board, December 2019.

SIGRID WECHT: *Cyril is not as difficult, blustering or angry as people may think. He is much kinder. He is a sweet, generous person. As the Israelis would say, he is a "sabra," a fruit that is prickly on the outside, but soft on the inside. His public persona is very different from his private one.*

SUSAN SHANAMAN: *Once, I was sitting at a meeting and a woman, who I didn't know, introduced herself to me. I mentioned that I worked for the coroners (in Pennsylvania) and she asked, "Do you know Cyril Wecht?" I said, "Yes, I do." Then she said, "He's just the most wonderful person in the world. When I was young," she continued, "I was growing up in Pittsburgh, and my mother died. Dr. Wecht [who was Allegheny County Coroner at the time] called to see if everything had been taken care of properly with regard to my mother. He took the time to call me, personally, to see if I was all right, and I will never forget that."*

DANIEL WECHT: *One day, I operated on a patient who had a brain tumor. She wasn't really all with it yet, but she said, "Can I ask you a question?" I said, "Absolutely." "You wouldn't, by chance, be related to the 'real' Dr. Wecht, would you?" I get some variation of that all the time.*

INGRID WECHT: *My dad has lived his life the way that suited him. A lot of people can't say that.*

DONALD GUTER: *Cyril is a celebrity, as much as anybody, but didn't leave his roots to become one. He didn't leave his hometown to be the coroner or medical examiner for a bigger city. He made it big from Pittsburgh.*

DAVID WECHT: *My dad is definitely a folk hero in this region. If he's walking down the street, passersby will stop and say "Hello," and drivers will toot their horns. It's always fun to watch.*

Even at age 89, I still find myself in the thick of things. In 2019, I was nominated by Pennsylvania Governor Tom Wolf to the state's Coroners' Education Board, and was approved by the State Senate in November. In December, my son David swore me in. And in Beaver County, the new Midland Innovation and Technology Charter School (MITCS), which is set to open its doors in the fall of 2020, has named an Academy for Forensics and Law after me.

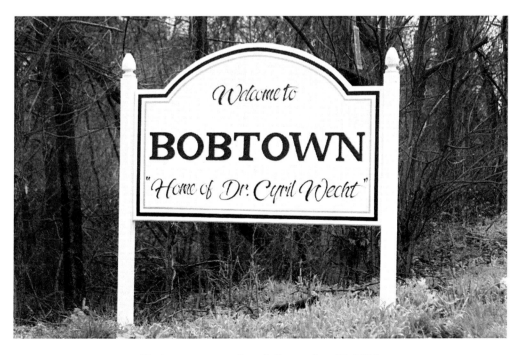

Native son remembered, September 25, 2016.

STEPHEN CATANZARITE: *At MITCS, we seek to work with and/or honor people from the western Pennsylvania region who have made great contributions to their fields. These figures include legendary composer Henry Mancini, Oscar-winning special effects artist Joe Letteri, post-pop artist Burton Morris, and jazz guitarist Joe Negri, to name a few. Working with the Wecht family and naming an Academy for Forensics and Law after Cyril is very much in that tradition. It is part and parcel of promoting our region and celebrating and continuing to build up the local community.*

Eight years ago, at the age of 81, I went "ziplining" in Norway, and dove from a cliff into an ice-cold Norwegian lake, demonstrating the patented swan dive I learned as a kid. This is nothing to boast of; it's something to be thankful for. Where my drive and energy come from, I can't tell you. But when it comes to living my life, as the late Frank Sinatra once sang, "I did it my way."

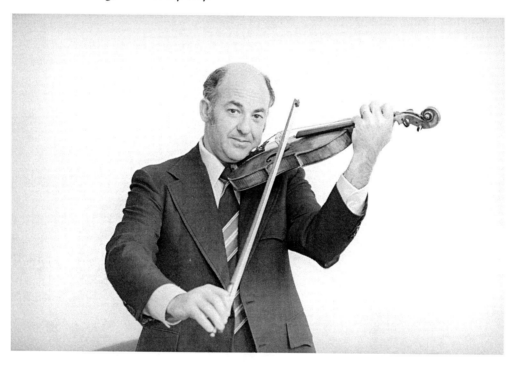

Still making music, after all these years (*Jim Judkis*).

The Cyril H. Wecht Institute of Forensic Science and Law

BEN WECHT: *Education has always been extremely important to my dad. He's been a member of multiple university faculties for decades, including Duquesne University's law and pharmacy schools. Among other pedagogical philosophies, he has always believed that if we're ever going to achieve greater social justice and enhanced public safety in this country, scientific and legal education must be joined together.*

Too many scientists and too many attorneys don't know what the other profession does, and yet they rely on each other so heavily. I can't tell you how many times I've heard lawyers in court discussing physical evidence about which they seemed to know little or nothing. As a result, neither did the judge nor the jury. So, I decided that I wanted to create an academic environment where scientists and lawyers could talk to and learn from each other.

KATHLEEN SEKULA: *I believe that Cyril first conceived this idea in the wake of the O.J. Simpson trial, in 1995. That trial, which was televised, captured the nation's imagination, and made it clear to Cyril that the law didn't understand science, and science didn't understand the law.*

JOHN RAGO: *For some of us, the outcome of the Simpson trial was insulting, yet it was also amazing, on many levels. Fresh on the heels of the verdict, Cyril had the idea to bring Henry Lee, Barry Scheck, and as many of the principles of the Simpson trial as possible to Duquesne University for a special program about the case.*

At the time, these players were like "rock stars," having been on television every day for months. So, when Cyril said that he'd like to bring them in, we all said, "How is that going to happen?" But Cyril did bring them all together as only Cyril could. He made phone calls and they all said, "Yes."

NICHOLAS CAFARDI: *I first met Cyril in 1993, when I was the new Dean of the Duquesne University School of Law. Cyril was teaching a course, as an adjunct, in "law and medicine," and he was a popular professor. The students liked him because of the personal experiences he brought to that course. Then one day, Cyril told me that he had this idea for an institute of forensic science and law. So, I brought the idea to a meeting of Duquesne's deans, and it had an electric effect.*

We designed an educational component in the form of a certificate program, and talked about it with several schools at Duquesne, saying, "We'd like to introduce the law to science and science to the law." And I wanted the world to see what forensic science could do for many other disciplines, too.

NICHOLAS CAFARDI: *The Dean of the School of Nursing said, "We could train nurses in forensic medicine." The Dean of Duquesne's School of Business said, "Forensic accounting is a really big thing these days." And the Dean of the School of Natural and Environmental Sciences added, "Forensics involves the kind of science we are teaching." So, I got buy-in from my fellow deans and from the academic vice president as well. Then the question became: "How do we do this?"*

I went back to Cyril and he made a generous gift to get things started, in return for which we named the institute after him. I want to make it clear that the naming was not a condition of the gift. When Cyril provided the money, he had no idea what the institute would be called.

In 2000, Duquesne's President, John E. Murray, Jr., adopted our plan, and the "Cyril H. Wecht Institute of Forensic Science and Law" was born. The seed was planted and the tree kept growing.

BEN WECHT: *My dad was the driving force from day one. He held meetings and bought everybody dinner, doing whatever it would take to get the train out of the station. Most academics think things through to the point where they kill an idea. But my dad is a "results guy." When he gets passionate, it's time for the talking to stop. It's time to get moving and act.*

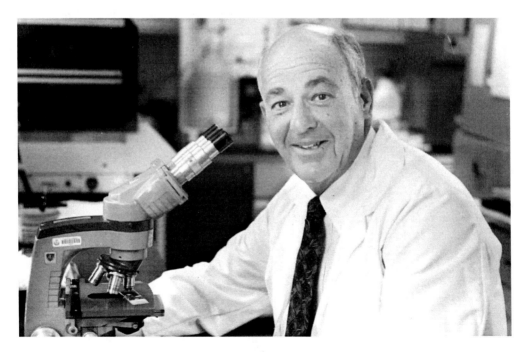

Allegheny County Coroner—again, 1998.

Early on, we had great success with the creation of the multi-disciplinary Certificate in Forensic Science and Law, a sort of survey course introducing students to the major forensic scientific disciplines, the fundamentals of criminal and civil law, and a handful of applications. Initially an exclusively on-site program, it attracted 70–75 students to our first class. We had perhaps 40 speakers come and go over the course of that first year—all brand-name folks. We later added a mock crime scene investigation, led by a former Pittsburgh police detective, and a mock trial, led by practicing attorneys and presided over by an active judge.

KEN GORMLEY: *Most recently, the Institute implemented a distance-learning option to its programming, making it available to a wider audience and enhancing Duquesne University's continuing reputation as an online education provider.*

KATHLEEN SEKULA: *If a student must relocate to accept a new position or, in the case of the military, if a student gets deployed, he or she can continue with our program via the Internet. Nurses apply to us from all over the nation, from foreign countries, and even from the U.S. military, because our program happens totally online.*

It's a stimulating, exciting course of study for people from all walks of life. Other universities became partners, and it has continued to play an important role for the community and for Duquesne. As an example, the relationship between the nursing school at Duquesne and the Wecht Institute has been a good one.

KATHLEEN SEKULA: *In 2002, we applied to the federal Health Resources and Services Administration (HRSA) and received a three-year grant for approximately $1.5 million. Collaborating with the Wecht Institute was really the strength of our proposal. It made us stand out. Subsequently, we received a continuation grant of $1.5 million from the HRSA for another three years. As a result, we were one of the very first universities to create a forensic master's program in nursing, and our program is growing all the time. It's a broad umbrella that covers all of the various areas in which forensic nurses might practice.*

What sets forensic nurses apart from other nurses is that they are trained to understand the legal implications that can present in a hospital or clinical setting regarding a victim, or even a perpetrator, of violence. They learn how to identify patients who may arrive with physical symptoms but have not revealed that they've been the victim of a crime. They learn how to do evidence collection in acute cases while the incident is still fresh, and much, much more.

JOHN RAGO: *Like all new programs, the Institute was, at the start, sort of organized chaos. We were creating something that didn't exist anywhere before, but we knew what we had to do to be successful. We had to bring the best people we could to Duquesne, and have the best kinds of conversations, discussions and classes. If we did that, we would inspire people to find a broader direction in their work. That was Cyril's vision because, while we couldn't produce a room full of forensic scientists, we could produce a nurse who was more in-tune with how to handle sexual assaults, or an insurance investigator who was more in-tune with suicide. Pick the industry and discipline and we could accentuate it.*

The Wecht Institute was conceived to host an annual conference that would attract national luminaries to talk about cases and issues that involve forensic science and law. In my estimation, the most remarkable to date was our program marking the 40th anniversary of the JFK assassination, which we put on in 2003. It was a real "who's who" of JFK experts and aficionados, including Oliver Stone, director of the film *JFK*, who would come back again 10 years later for our program on the assassination's 50th anniversary.

DONALD GUTER: *I was Dean of the Duquesne University School of Law from 2005 through the end of 2008, and have seen many college and law school programs in my day, but Cyril's Institute programs were real extravaganzas. He could call on anyone and they would show up. You would have to be an isolated person who was not interested in anything to not have an appreciation for his programs, or to attend one of them and not learn something.*

KEN GORMLEY: *The Institute's annual symposium and other continuing education programs are among the best in the region. They've drawn experts, scholars, and legal and medical professionals to share their experiences, expertise and stories with other professionals and members of the public who want to learn more about the fascinating and far-reaching field of forensic science.*

We seeded and nurtured a five-year, entry-level master's degree program in forensic science and law in which students take two or three very rigorous years of chemistry, biology and math, among other subjects, with courses in such areas of American legal history, torts and ethics entering in the fourth year. In that program, which is closely affiliated with the Wecht Institute and now co-housed in the Bayer School of Natural and Environmental Sciences, we offer students not just the underpinning of forensic scientific practice, but practical applications for what they're learning and a sense of why it's important. We talk to them about their need to be fiercely independent because they will be working for one client in the end—the truth.

I'm proud of the fact that we've been able to set many people on course for greater effectiveness in their professional lives. But the work of the Institute goes well beyond my personal legacy, straight into the heart of justice in our society. We want to make sure that prosecutions are not undertaken for political reasons, and that people are not wrongfully convicted. If the police are involved in a homicide, we believe that it must be revealed. Many other scenarios exist in which, historically, justice has not prevailed. The process begins with lawyers and continues through scientific experts. How much they collaborate is the key to better and more just legal outcomes.

BEN WECHT: *What's important is that people who are practicing in the fields of science and law are better at their jobs when they learn what we teach them. And it's not just applications. It's ethics. It's values. And it's the pursuit of truth. That's what drives my dad. I don't care if you're a scientist, field investigator, lawyer, nurse or accountant, there are people whose focus has been changed substantially, and maybe indelibly, because of my dad and what he has done.*

Through the years, I've connected with Duquesne law students, science students, psychology students, and so on. It has been a pleasure for me, and I don't intend to quit now. I'm always ready to go. It would take a conscious effort of the highest magnitude to stifle my passion.

JOHN RAGO: *Cyril is such an inspirational, high-energy person. Sometimes I worry about his workload, but I've seen no sign of abatement. He seems to be able to keep going and going.*

BEN WECHT: *The Cyril H. Wecht Institute of Forensic Science and Law today is almost completely registration-based. Today, our income is generated mostly via professional and general public registration for the programs that we put on. In the Continuing Legal Education market, there is a huge amount of competition, including other online providers. But we're now building up our archival offerings so that we can, essentially, offer a menu of accredited material for people to purchase and view at their leisure, wherever they are. And we're pleased to report that, after a several-year hiatus, we are now back into academic programming, providing content for undergraduate and graduate-level seminars in the Master's of Forensic Science and Law program.*

I've made it a point to be generous to Duquesne University for helping me to maintain the Institute, and have redirected a lot of funding to the school. I give speaking engagements and ask the hosts to send my checks to Duquesne. That's routine for me. And when it comes to my legacy in the academic arena, there's no disputing that I'm well-established, which means a lot to me.

KEN GORMLEY: *After two decades, the Cyril H. Wecht Institute of Forensic Science and Law remains relevant because it provides invaluable opportunities for professionals to stay up to date on current developments in forensic science and related subjects, while also providing the general public with a glimpse into the workings of this important field.*

Witness for Truth
Casework

As a forensic pathologist for nearly 60 years, I've been involved in thousands of diverse cases: from local and national to international; and from civil proceedings to high-profile criminal cases. In my view, all cases, especially those that result in death, are important, no matter the victim or the perpetrator.

ALAN DERSHOWITZ: *I've tried more than 30 homicide cases during my career and won almost all of them by using forensic science evidence, the kind of material that Cyril has been gathering and analyzing for many years. I taught my students [at Harvard] that, to become good lawyers, they must be knowledgeable about a range of scientific issues. Cyril was, in many ways, the originator. He was the first name that I knew when I started teaching and practicing in the area of law and science. Our paths have crossed dozens of times, but I knew his work well before I met him.*

As you've come to know, I have always been an active and involved person. I am proud to say that, at one time or another in my career, I was president of the two largest organizations in my field: the American College of Legal Medicine, and the American Academy of Forensic Sciences. I was a charter diplomate and the first chairman of the American Board of Legal Medicine, and a charter diplomate and the first vice-president of the American Board of Disaster Medicine. In 1965, I was instrumental in founding the Pittsburgh Institute of Legal Medicine. Members of this non-profit group received our quarterly publication called *Scalpel and Quill*, and opportunities to attend the international conferences we hosted every year for three decades throughout the U.S., Europe, South America, Africa, the Caribbean, China and Hong Kong. We also offered domestic programs to our membership led by top-level professionals including several department-oriented chairs at the University of Pittsburgh School of Medicine.

To date, I have published eight true crime books about famous and fascinating cases, in many of which I had been involved, directly or indirectly. For the public, these cases hold a special interest, and when people hear me speak about them—on television, radio, or from the podium—they are tremendously interested and enthusiastic. People seem to revel in gaining a view from the "inside" of famous and sensational cases, and are eager to get my take on them.

Donnie Eichar: *I read Dr. Wecht's book,* Mortal Evidence, *and there was one case in there about a guy who tortured his victims by putting cement in their ears and Drāno in their eyes. I read about that case around lunchtime one day and, afterward, I had to go for a long walk because it disturbed me so much. I had never heard of anything so awful. I talked to Dr. Wecht about it later and asked him, "How do you deal with this kind of stuff? How do you let it go?"*

◆ ◆ ◆

Ronald Freeman: *I was a police officer in Pittsburgh for more than 37 years. As a homicide detective, I was involved with Dr. Wecht on a professional level and, over time, as a friend, when he was the Coroner of Allegheny County.*

In addition to being a forensic scientist, Cyril was a teacher, and that's what attracted me to him, initially. When I went to the scene of a homicide, I wanted to know as much as I could about the bodies of the victims and the way they reacted to certain things. I also wanted to know about what to consider when investigating such cases, and what to look for.

Cyril always took the time to talk with us about individual cases and would answer any questions that we had. What we learned from one case would carry over to others. But not only would he do that, he would also offer seminars for homicide investigators, which was ultimately to the benefit of the police as a whole, and the people we served.

Roy Kirk

Pittsburgh is not really a big city, yet I have conducted much of my work here and have dealt with many strange and peculiar cases. Consider the 1997 case of Roy Kirk, and its grisly trappings.

Roy Kirk and Ann Hoover both owned properties on Lawn Street, in the South Oakland section of Pittsburgh, where residents were trying to gentrify the neighborhood in a bid to raise the value of what they owned. But Mr. Kirk did not properly maintain several properties that he owned there, which included a crumbling, abandoned rowhouse, the poor state of which led to water damage on the properties located on either side of it.

One of the contiguous properties that had sustained water damage was owned by Ms. Hoover, who had asked Mr. Kirk many times to renovate the properties he owned in the neighborhood, but he had always refused. So, when Kirk failed to come up with the funds needed to repair his rowhouse, Hoover and other neighbors took him to housing court.

One day, a hearing was scheduled for that suit, but neither Kirk nor Hoover appeared. Concerned, Hoover's family asked the police to do a "welfare check," and officers were dispatched to her home. When they pulled up and knocked on Hoover's door, they received no answer, so they went to Kirk's abandoned property next door and did likewise, with the same result. Kirk's door, however, was left ajar, so the officers entered cautiously only to discover, in the basement, Roy Kirk dismembering the body of 44-year-old Ann Hoover, with hand and circular saws.

Kirk's rowhouse was adjoined to Hoover's so, after he killed her, of which there was no doubt, he dragged her body to his place through a tunnel he had dug in his basement wall, and began cutting-up her body to dispose of it, in an effort to cover his tracks. Of course, the police officers on the scene arrested Mr. Kirk, placed him in handcuffs with his hands behind his back, and put him into a police wagon. All the while, Kirk was screaming and imploring the police to kill him.

RONALD FREEMAN: *Mr. Kirk was in the wagon, and it's significant that he was handcuffed behind his back. Homicide detectives, including me, had arrived and were advised as to what was discovered, so I told the officers to transport Kirk to our offices so that he could be interviewed. The wagon then drove to our building and, when it arrived and the officers opened the doors, Roy Kirk was found dead inside. Apparently, he had used his belt and hanged himself. When I saw this, I thought, "Who will ever believe that a prisoner who was handcuffed behind his back could hang himself in a police vehicle all on his own with his own belt?" I knew that the only way we were going to survive this turn of events [and the negative media attention that would certainly have followed] was if Cyril Wecht believed us, so I called him up, saying, "Cyril, I need you here right now." "Why?" he asked. So, I told him, and, "boom," he came right away.*

Ron briefed me on what had happened and I interviewed the two officers who transported Roy Kirk. "Were they the kind of police officers who would deliberately kill a person?" Next, the officers opened the wagon and I inspected it, after which I instructed them to summon someone from the Crime Lab who was about the same height and weight as Mr. Kirk. When that person arrived, we handcuffed him behind his back and placed him in the police wagon. Was it possible for Roy Kirk to have removed his belt and hanged himself so quickly in such a situation? It was. We timed it multiple times and determined that it could be done in less than three minutes. I determined that his death was a suicide and not due to actions on the part of the police officers.

◆ ◆ ◆

F. LEE BAILEY: *In many trials, defense attorneys are presented with a dilemma. Would you rather have the testimony of a "prince among men" who doesn't speak very well, or that of a bright and maybe not-quite-so-sincere expert who can tell a good story? The answer is that most lawyers would rather have the latter because it's more persuasive. Cyril fits both bills. He is a bright and honest guy who knows the science, and he is extremely articulate. He's also a lawyer and has good insight when it comes to any bag of tricks that attorneys might use to try to discredit him. So, if something is afoot by way of a "sucker question," Cyril can see it coming.*

ALAN DERSHOWITZ: *There's no such thing as a "good" forensic expert witness. There are only good scientists who can communicate their science on the stand. I think the fact that Cyril is also a lawyer helps, but the fact that he's a good scientist who leaves no stone unturned is what makes him so imposing on the stand. Cyril is good on the stand because he's good before he gets on the stand. He has tremendous credibility.*

F. LEE BAILEY: *I've never seen anybody get ahead of Cyril on the witness stand, and I would not want to see him on the other side of my cases, unless I had something in my back pocket that would fly in the face of his diagnosis, because he's likely to be believed.*

My take on the case of Charles Dixon, the black man who had succumbed from positional asphyxiation at the hands of police officers in Pittsburgh, nearly led me to ruin, financially and otherwise, in federal court. My independence and dogged pursuit of the truth left me exposed in Pittsburgh and Allegheny County, especially when it came to cases involving the police. But when it came to national cases, I was free to offer my views without hassles from local detractors. For the purposes of brevity, I will offer my opinions on a number of cases that you likely will know, and about which much has been said, on TV and in books. I didn't create the controversies that surrounded these cases. They came with baggage all their own.

High-Profile Cases

The first thing you must know is that, when a case reaches the point of national notoriety, frankly, the attorneys on both sides become enthralled. And I don't care what their own personal ambitions may be; everybody loves the spotlight. In high-profile cases with lots of media attention, lawyers will milk those situations for all they're worth. And they'll want to make sure that they don't "blow it"—especially the prosecution—by not covering every single detail. So, testimony will often be repetitive and excessive and, sometimes, foolishly and mistakenly so.

High-profile cases involving homicide garner the most attention, and questions about murder have been posed to me thousands of times over the years. They're asked every day by the "man on the street" and even by professionals like me, who deal with the bodies of the victims. There are crimes that we will never accept, rationalize or justify or, in any way, attempt to ameliorate, but which we can fully understand. But there are others. Some killers are truly evil. Sometimes, they're mentally deranged. But a large percentage of murders and murderers are inexplicable.

I don't go seeking cases. Most often, people reach out to me, or my involvement comes about indirectly through the news media. The case involving the death of Elvis Presley came by way of an inquiry from ABC's "20/20" program, for example. For Robert Kennedy, my old friend and now former Chief Medical Examiner of Los Angeles County, Dr. Thomas Noguchi, called me. F. Lee Bailey recommended me to the DA of Suffolk County for the Chappaquiddick case involving U.S. Senator Ted Kennedy. And prominent attorney Mark Geragos contacted me about Scott Peterson. So, I don't hustle business, not that there's anything wrong with that. And I'm not saying this because I want to make myself seem "purer-than-thou," but I don't advertise. Nonetheless, I get cases from all over.

HENRY LEE: *I've known Cyril for 30 or 40 years now. I am in criminalistics, and I'm pretty good at it. But he's a leader in forensic pathology. We sometimes work on cases together and that's how we became friends. We've worked together on some high-profile ones, and we respect each other very much. Some people think that Cyril is too controversial, but I don't.*

JonBenét Ramsey

In 1996, on Christmas Day, six-year-old JonBenét Ramsey, a child beauty queen, was killed in her family's home in Boulder, Colorado. The cause of death was determined to be asphyxia by strangulation with craniocerebral trauma. I was away in the Caribbean when I got a call from the *National Enquirer* asking if I would take a look at some pictures of a little girl. The story hadn't yet broken in the *New York Times*, and I didn't know who she was. But I remember noticing the girl's makeup and comportment, and how strange it all seemed. Things evolved from there.

My belief is that little JonBenét died during some sort of sex game perpetrated by her father, John Ramsey. I don't think that there was intent to harm her, let alone kill her, but I am aware of such games wherein a rope is tied around a female's neck and the vagina is penetrated, in this case likely with a finger not a penis. When you constrict someone's neck, the person gets what is called a "vagal reflex" that can lead to cardiac arrhythmia and sudden death.

Early on, the local DA, who rarely pursued a case to trial, cleared JonBenét's parents, John and Patsy Ramsey, of any connection to the death of their daughter. How could they have lived with themselves if the truth had come out? I guess they made a decision: "JonBenét is gone, and we'll grieve, but we just can't tell this story."

The case was a mess from the start. The investigators were totally incompetent, and their bias led to manipulation by the little girl's wealthy parents. On top of that, the local district attorney was wholly inadequate, and that sealed the deal for injustice. But in my view, the greater injustice had to do with social inequity. The Ramseys, with the support of prominent and well-connected lawyers, were never interrogated separately and fully. I have no doubt that if this case had evolved in a family of lower socioeconomic status, it would not have gone unsolved.

I see cases all the time that are the antithesis of this one, where people are accused of child abuse and the charges are overstated. Prosecutors come on like gangbusters against the parents but, when it came to the Ramseys, they treated them with kid gloves. One of their high-powered attorneys from Atlanta actually threatened to sue me for some of the things I was saying in the press. The Ramseys were retaliating: "We're going to bring a defamation action against anybody who suggests that we had anything to do with this." But the lawyer backed off when I told him to go screw himself. The Ramseys attacked and threatened everybody, but I called their bluff.

The JonBenét Ramsey case was a travesty of justice. There may have been no murder, but it was certainly manslaughter, and if you wanted to raise it to second-degree because of the child sexual abuse, that might have been appropriate. No intruder entered the Ramseys' home and killed JonBenét. The evidence does not support that.

HENRY LEE: *I don't think that JonBenét's death was a homicide. I think it was a family tragedy and the mother tried to cover it up, so it was staged like a homicide. Remember the ransom note? "We are a small group of foreign terrorists..." No terrorist group is going to call itself "small," even if there were only two members. Then think about such a group asking for only $118,000. Why not ask for more? The ransom note was three pages long.*

No terrorist would write that much, and leave two practice notes in a nearby trash can, from the same notepad.

Claus von Bülow

In late 1980, Danish-British socialite Claus von Bülow's wife, Sunny, lay in a deep coma. Prosecutors claimed that her condition was due to an overdose of certain drugs that had been administered to her by her husband.

Claus von Bülow's 1982 trial was bungled by his defense counsel, William Fallon, an attorney from Buffalo who, although quite experienced, never bothered to seek the input of forensic science experts, even though forensic science evidence was the crux of the case. Claus was found "guilty" and sentenced to 30 years in prison. The verdict, however, was overturned on appeal.

The second time around, in 1985, von Bülow was represented by Alan Dershowitz, one of the foremost attorneys in the country. Dershowitz, who is a friend of mine, was a professor of law at Harvard, a distinguished writer and lecturer, and a brilliant intellect. Alan got involved with the retrial, along with Tom Puccio, formerly a prominent federal prosecutor whose accomplishments included several ABSCAM convictions. (ABSCAM was an FBI sting operation in the late 1970s and early 1980s that led to the convictions of seven members of the U.S. Congress, among others.)

Dershowitz and Puccio contacted me, forensic pathologist Michael Baden, a top-notch forensic toxicologist and a top-notch pharmacologist, and we had some spirited meetings about the facts of the case. I remember attending a dinner at von Bülow's beautiful Fifth Avenue apartment in New York to review things. At von Bülow's retrial, Dershowitz and Puccio did a great job of showing that there was no evidence at all to prove that Claus had done anything to cause his wife's coma.

Sunny von Bülow exhibited all the signs of suffering from what is called "polypharmacy," meaning that she maintained, in her bedroom and bathroom, a collection of pills and medicines that would have rivaled some drugstores. Aspirin, painkillers, anti-depressants, tranquilizers: whatever kind of drug she thought she needed to treat her various maladies (real or imagined), she had it. Sunny was taking all kinds of drugs and wound up all but killing herself in the process.

In the retrial, defense experts testified that the hypodermic needle—tainted with insulin, but on the outside only—had been dipped in insulin, but could not have been injected. (After stabbing it into the flesh, the withdrawal of the needle would have wiped the outside of it clean.) Defense evidence also showed that, when Sunny von Bülow was admitted to the hospital three weeks before the onset of her coma, she had ingested at least 73 aspirin tablets, a quantity that could only have been self-administered. This fact clearly demonstrated that Sunny von Bülow's state-of-mind was indeed fragile at the time of the incident in question. In the end, the testimony of several of the experts Alan had called upon showed that there was no basis to prove that Claus von Bülow caused his wife's coma, and Claus was acquitted.

To this day, I believe that Sunny's children by her first marriage, Annie-Laurie von Auersperg and Alexander-Georg von Auersperg, attempted to frame their stepfather for what amounted to an accident. There was antipathy, and it was all related to inheritance, but the matter was resolved over time. The daughter of Claus and Sunny von Bülow, Cosima, got her share of Sunny's estate, and Sunny's children from her previous marriage got theirs. Claus moved from the U.S. to England, and I continued a correspondence with him for some time. He died in London on May 25, 2019, at age 92. (Sunny von Bülow remained in a persistent vegetative state for 28 years, until her death from cardiopulmonary arrest on December 6, 2008.)

Can I rule out the possibility that Claus von Bülow may have deliberately encouraged his wife to take certain drugs? No. But one shouldn't base a murder case on conjecture alone, or because of what one may think about the individuals involved. You must have proof, and there was no proof that Claus had given Sunny any particular drug. There was evidence, however, that she had been using certain drugs all by herself, and the drugs that were found in her system, by way of toxicological analysis, all comported with what she was known to have taken many times before.

When you think about it, deaths due to acute combined drug toxicity are not rare. When two, four, six, eight or 10 drugs work together to depress the central nervous system, the end result is respiratory depression, followed by cardiac arrhythmia. The brain is insulted from a lack of oxygen because the lungs and heart aren't working. Finally, the brain's control over the heart and lungs diminishes, the lungs finally surrender, and the person goes into cardio-respiratory arrest.

In my estimation, the Claus von Bülow verdict, in the end, was a just one. But the case still bothers me from the standpoint of professionalism. How could an experienced attorney like William Fallon, who I'm sure was paid a substantial sum of money for his efforts, totally miss the boat?

The Branch Davidians

Between February 28 and April 19, 1993, a compound belonging to the Branch Davidian religious sect was under siege by American federal and Texas state law enforcement, as well as the U.S. military. The Branch Davidians were led by a man named David Koresh, and were headquartered at Mount Carmel Center ranch in the community of Axtell, Texas, 13 miles east of Waco.

Suspecting that the group was stockpiling illegal weapons, the Bureau of Alcohol, Tobacco and Firearms (ATF) obtained a search warrant for the compound and arrest warrants for Koresh and several of the group's members. When the ATF attempted to raid the ranch, a gun battle erupted, resulting in the deaths of four government agents and six Branch Davidians.

Given the ATF's failure in that raid, a siege was undertaken by the government that lasted 51 days and culminated with a tear-gas assault by the FBI in an attempt to force the Branch Davidians to flee the compound. But during the attack, a fire engulfed Mount Carmel Center. In total, 76 people died, including Koresh. And quite uncharacteristically, I went after this case. I contacted the attorney for David Koresh, and he immediately accepted my help.

I conducted autopsies on Koresh and his two top associates, and reviewed the autopsy findings of other deceased Davidian members. By way of that process, I showed that none had committed suicide during the conflagration, as had been alleged by the Feds. Many had multiple gunshot wounds and were alive for a time, at least, while the fire was raging. I also showed, in essence, using forensic scientific evidence, that the attack was initiated by the Feds (the ATF and FBI), and raised questions about the gunshot wounds. (All of this came out during civil actions against the federal government that resulted in substantial settlements for the victims.)

At the outset, the ATF and FBI said that all the shots had come from within the Davidian's compound. The results of my autopsies, correlated with other known facts about the raid and its outcome, showed this simply wasn't true. We also discovered that the Feds knew, somehow, that David Koresh had learned of their plans to assault the compound. I guess they figured they had better get the drop on him and strike first.

I'm not sure what the alleged crimes of the Branch Davidians were exactly—technical violations regarding firearms, I think—but they hadn't, to my knowledge, hurt or threatened anyone. The Feds also expressed concerns about allegations that the children who lived with their parents within the compound were being abused. So, let's get this straight: The government knew that there was likely going to be an armed conflict; and they also knew that children were present. Why risk the lives of the innocent? After all, the government knew that Koresh, from time to time, left the compound to make purchases for himself and his followers. Why didn't the Feds just arrest him on the street in town if he had broken the law? Why did they let him return home and then storm the compound? Eventually, the Davidians would have run out of food and water. Why not arrest them at that time, peacefully? Why? Because that's not how the ATF or FBI work.

I recall a case in the Pittsburgh area, in Indiana Township, where the FBI smashed in a person's door at 3 or 4 a.m., and the woman who lived there shot and killed an FBI agent. She was aware that her husband was involved in some shady dealings, but all she knew at the time was that somebody was smashing-in her door, and she and her kids were scared. I also remember what the FBI did in Bellevue, a suburb of Pittsburgh, to a local black family. They smashed in their door looking for a woman who hadn't been there in two years (which the FBI should have known). In the middle of the night, they forced the frightened occupants of the residence to get down on the floor, and then made them go outside, half-naked. These are Gestapo tactics, my friends.

I am disturbed by the FBI and its quasi-fascistic history, and also by the U.S. Supreme Court, which has decided to allow federal agents to move ahead without warrants in too many situations. The FBI is a powerful and dangerous organization—the legacy of the despicable J. Edgar Hoover—and it is becoming more and more of an unrestrained national police force. It is fascinating to note how the public's perception of the FBI has changed as a result of the Robert Mueller probe and other investigations related to President Donald Trump.

O.J. Simpson

Anyone who was alive in 1995 knows about the O.J. Simpson case, the criminal trial which was held at the Los Angeles County Superior Court. Former National Football League hero, sports broadcaster and occasional actor O.J. Simpson was tried on two counts of murder for the June 12, 1994, slashing deaths of his ex-wife, Nicole Brown Simpson, and her friend, Ronald Goldman.

F. LEE BAILEY: *I had sought to get Cyril involved with O.J. However, before I entered the case, Robert Shapiro had already called in Michael Baden, who is a very capable forensic pathologist in his own right. When I suggested that two forensic pathologists might be better than one, and that I thought we should still bring Cyril in, I received two responses: One: "You and Cyril are too close and the prosecution might have a lot of fun with that"; and two: "Cyril has already given quite a few opinions about the case to the press, so he wouldn't be coming in impartial." But I would have brought Cyril in anyway. He is always a successful witness.*

Lee Bailey's cross-examination of Mark Fuhrman in the O.J. Simpson trial should be compulsory study for every law student in America. To paraphrase: "Detective Fuhrman, as you sit here today, under oath, are you saying to His Honor, Judge Ito, and to the ladies and gentlemen of the jury, that you have never used the 'N'-word?" It had been documented that Fuhrman had used that word more than once on the job, and that he had been disciplined for it. But the prosecutors, Marcia Clark and Chris Darden, presumably knowing this, called Fuhrman anyway. If the defense had found out about Fuhrman's history, how could the prosecution not have known? And thanks to Lee Bailey, the jury was to know it, too.

I was consulted by the defense attorneys who were handling the case—Johnnie Cochran, Bob Shapiro, Lee Bailey and Barry Scheck—and worked with them and with other experts in my field, namely Michael Baden, and Henry Lee. In fact, Lee Bailey came to my home for a day or so to go over everything. I wound up not testifying, primarily because I had become such a frequent commentator about the case on national TV, but I worked on the case all the way through.

As for the verdict, I was in my office when the jury came in. People were saying, "He's guilty as hell." But I said, "He's going to be acquitted." Johnnie Cochran, Lee Bailey and Barry Scheck had done a tremendous job, from Lee's cross-examination of Fuhrman to getting into evidence the supposed "blood-soaked glove." More important, by having the case moved out of toney Brentwood to downtown L.A. the defense picked up a predominantly African American jury. Nine black people, along with one Hispanic person and two whites, sat in that jury box. What do you suppose they were thinking?

The case got screwed up by the authorities from the very beginning. The medical examiner was never called to the crime scene and the bodies were not examined by a forensic pathologist for more than 12 hours. Rigor mortis (body stiffening), livor mortis (gravitational settling of the blood in the dependent parts of the body), and algor mortis (body temperature), are the criteria we use to try to determine time of death. These are not scientifically precise, and the more time that elapses following a death, the more imprecise they become. So, when you talk about waiting until 12 hours after death, the ability to narrow things down to a tight timeframe is lost. That was key to the case because of the very small window of opportunity that O.J. Simpson had before he caught a plane and flew out of town on the night of the killings.

In the trial, a lot of interesting things played out. My old friend, Henry Lee, saw the blood-soaked glove that had been discovered by Mark Fuhrman after Fuhrman (inadvisably) climbed over a wall onto O.J.'s property. Even with Henry's relatively small hand, he couldn't get the glove to fit. So, Cochran said to the prosecution, "If you don't put that glove into evidence, we're going to do it." The prosecution, I guess, hadn't thought too much about it, so they put the glove into evidence. And before long, Johnnie Cochran was saying, "If it doesn't fit, you must acquit."

Was there absolutely no evidence suggesting that O.J. had committed the murders? Evidence was present, but it was all circumstantial. The prosecution did not have any "hard proof." And other questions remained of a forensic-scientific nature that were quite interesting.

Nicole Simpson and Ron Goldman sustained multiple stab wounds. These involved the neck area, including major vessels. When you sever a neck vessel—the carotid artery or the jugular vein—you get a significant spurting of blood. Remember, the victims were both young, healthy people. Their blood pressure would have been elevated as they fought for their lives, and their blood would have splashed all over. So, where was all the blood? The police never found it. But they did find one drop on O.J.'s sock. The problem was that the lead detective had collected 8-ccs of blood at the scene, which was documented by the medical technician—about a teaspoon-and-a-half—and carried it around in his pocket, something he admitted he had never done before; and he didn't turn it in for eight hours. When he did, it was logged in as containing 6.5-ccs. So, 1.5-ccs of blood was missing, more than enough to make a drop and place it anywhere.

Also interesting was the fact that Nicole Simpson had bloodstains on her back, which were never tested. If the medical examiner's office had done its job, if the prosecution had tested those stains, and if the tests had showed that the blood came from somebody other than O.J. Simpson, that would have been the end of the case. Maybe that's why the authorities didn't risk testing it.

Finally, the forensic pathologist who did the autopsies and testified at the preliminary hearing did such a terrible and embarrassing job that the prosecution didn't call him at trial. In fact, at the beginning of its case, the prosecution called the chief medical examiner, who had never even seen the bodies and did not participate in the autopsies, and had him acknowledge that his office had made 43 errors in the handling of the bodies and evidence. The prosecution knew, of course, that the defense team was aware of this, so they thought they better get it all out right away.

Whether O.J. Simpson was guilty or not, I can't say for sure. But I do believe this: He could not have committed both of those murders, inflicting all of those wounds on those two people, by himself, and been able to get rid of all the blood, the bloody clothing, and the murder weapon. The police examined the sink drains, toilet drains, showers, and bathtubs at O.J.'s home and found no evidence of blood, and blood is extremely sensitive to chemical testing. Where, then, did O.J. go to wash off the blood? Imagine the distance and the pathways between where the murders took place and where O.J. lived. That area was scoured for evidence, inch-by-inch. Every possible route that he might have taken was examined and studied in a most minute fashion, and the detectives never found anything. So, you have to ask yourself, "How was that possible?"

MICHAEL BADEN: *I testified at the O.J. Simpson trial. The evidence that was given for O.J. was not sufficient to say that he was the guilty person. Certainly, there are other people, perhaps close to O.J., who could have done it, but I didn't testify about who "might" have done it.*

My opinion is that the number of wounds, the struggle that took place, the energy that would have been expended, and the amount of blood that would have been spattered about, all point to a murder committed by more than one person. So, who might have assisted O.J. Simpson in the murder of his ex-wife and her friend? Someone very close to O.J., without a doubt.

Private investigator William C. Dear, in his book, *O.J. Is Innocent and I Can Prove It*, published in 2012, points to O.J. Simpson's elder son from his first marriage, Jason Simpson, as an obvious but overlooked suspect. Dear conducted more than 16 years of investigation and stated that it wasn't O.J. who killed Nicole Brown Simpson and Ronald Goldman on the night of June 12, 1994. It was Jason—alone. While I concur with William Dear that young Mr. Simpson might likely have been involved, personally, I believe that O.J. was at the scene, too. The cops, however, made a premature decision to zero-in on O.J. Simpson solely, ran with that, and thus blew the case.

GERALDO RIVERA: *It seems to me that Cyril's been around for most of my television career, and he's as great on TV as he is on the witness stand. He's got that kind of idiosyncratic charm that just comes across. I've had him on my shows many times, like for the case of JonBenét Ramsey, which is still unsolved. We also followed the O.J. Simpson trial together. Cyril played a role in analyzing the forensic evidence for us on "Rivera Live" during that sensational, televised saga. I thought he had that case exactly right.*

Scott Peterson

Scott Peterson sits today on death row at San Quentin State Prison for the murder of his wife, Laci, and their unborn child, whom the couple had planned to name "Conner."

Peterson had reported his pregnant wife missing on December 24, 2002, a day on which he first claimed to have been golfing and, later, said that he had gone fishing at the Berkeley Marina, about 90 miles from the couple's home in Modesto, California. Scott Peterson had a history of extra-marital affairs with women, the last one of which he told that he had "lost his wife"—14 days before Laci disappeared.

MARK GERAGOS: *I consulted with Cyril over the years on various cases, most notably on Scott Peterson. We went to Modesto together, to the scene of Laci's disappearance. That's where I first saw the interplay between Cyril and Henry Lee, as Cyril consulted with him regarding the scene at the Peterson house. To me, their friendship is magical. The amount of knowledge that the two of them have and the depth of their experience is just incredible. And when I witnessed the interplay between them, it was hard to ever have anything but a smile on my face.*

I was contacted by Mark Geragos and went out to do a second autopsy on Laci Peterson. Henry Lee was with me, and we went to the place where the boat that Scott allegedly used to dump his wife's body in the Berkeley Marina was docked, and then on to the Peterson house, where we had to climb over a high fence because the entrance was blocked off.

I did repeat autopsies on Laci and Conner. Unfortunately, Laci's remains were so decomposed that nothing could be ascertained. As a matter of fact, there was not much left of her: no head and no arms; one leg was missing; only part of another leg remained; and her internal organs were gone. The only thing that remained was her uterus. But baby Conner's body was intact, and I thought, "Maybe there is a chance that I could determine whether or not he had been born alive." But although intact, Conner's organs were also in such an advanced state of decomposition that a microscopic examination of his lungs would have been meaningless.

MARK GERAGOS: *Cyril looks at things from a perspective that is invaluable. His experience, plus the fact that he is trained as a lawyer means that he understands what I'm looking for. What kinds of things can be potentially admissible? What is speculation and what is not speculation? He is one of the top five people in his field, anywhere in the world, and he's one of the hardest workers I know. I can reach him at any time, day or night, weekdays and weekends.*

Sometime later, Henry happened to be at my home in Pittsburgh. We were to fly out together on a Sunday to meet with Mark Geragos and testify in the Scott Peterson case the next day. Thinking about the situation, I said to Henry, "We can't give Mark anything more than he already has from the forensic pathologist who did the original autopsy," who said that he couldn't determine when, where or how Laci Peterson had died, because of the absence of tissues to examine. I had reviewed his testimony, and we helped Mark prepare for cross-examination. Sure enough, Mark got everything that he would have gotten from me on direct, as his witness. Why give the prosecution a chance to go through everything again with Henry and me, and remind the jury of what a heinous crime had been committed? So, I called Mark and, because he's such an intelligent attorney, he appreciated what I was saying, and agreed. I'm proud of the fact that, even on cases for which I'd not only be making significant money, but getting a lot of news coverage, too, if I don't think I can help, I don't hesitate to say so.

At some of my public-speaking engagements, when I reiterate that we could not determine the time, place or mechanism of Laci Peterson's death, people are often shocked. Fortunately, the circumstantial evidence in the case against Scott Peterson was so overwhelming that it did not make any difference. The point I want to make is that, today in the U.S., one can not only convict somebody of first-degree murder without having the victim's body, one can convict somebody of first-degree murder without even having "direct evidence."

I think the "guilty" verdict in the Scott Peterson case was correct, based upon the circumstantial evidence alone. If that jury could have come out of the jury box, they would have lynched him in the courtroom. They hated him so much, and said so shortly after the verdict was handed down. It's the way some defendants come across. Sometimes they arouse sympathy. But Scott Peterson, for a variety of reasons, did not gain the least bit of sympathy from those jurors.

HENRY LEE: *Scott Peterson basically convicted himself. The trouble is they had recordings of him. His wife had just died and he was talking to his girlfriend. The jury didn't need anything else.*

The Menendez Brothers

There's no question that the Menendez brothers, Lyle and Erik, shot and killed their parents premeditatedly in August of 1989. After shooting José and Kitty Menendez with shotguns while the couple sat watching television, the boys went outside, reloaded their guns, and came back for more.

The Menendez brothers were arrested in 1990 for the killings and, in 1993, were tried separately by different juries. Each claimed "self defense" due to years of alleged abuse at the hands of both parents. Both juries were "hung," so mistrials were declared. But the brothers were tried again together before a single jury in 1995. The goal of their attorneys during the retrial was to get not only physical abuse allegations into evidence, but sexual abuse as well.

I came aboard for that retrial and do believe that there had been some sexual abuse of the younger brother by the father. This didn't justify Erik's killing him but, at least, it hinted at a plausible reason for the murders. Why did the boys shoot their mother? Because she knew about the sexual abuse and never made a move to stop it, I suppose.

In the initial trials, almost amazingly, the juries were hung in what I thought should have been slam-dunk cases. The Los Angeles prosecutors were embarrassed (as well they should have been). The second time around, determined not to fail again, they hired an outfit called Failure Analysis Associates (FAA), a very reputable firm (which now goes by the name "Exponent").

FAA was an American engineering and scientific consulting firm with a multidisciplinary team of scientists, physicists, engineers and business consultants who were ready and able to do research and analysis in more than 90 technical disciplines. The boss there at the time, Roger McCarthy, hates me, and you'll soon learn why.

FAA had 50 or more highly educated people with whom to consult about the Menendez case, and the prosecution spent more than $1 million on their services—and this was 25 years ago. Roger McCarthy testified for seven-and-a-half days about what was, essentially, a case of four people and two shotguns in a small, darkened room, with the only light emanating from a television screen. He presented a scenario, with "reasonable scientific certainty," outlining the sequence of the 14 shotgun blasts, and the exact positions of each of the four people in the room for each shot.

I testified for less than half-a-day, and simply explained that, if a person was being shot at, he or she would be ducking, twisting, turning, jumping, leaping and then, ultimately, falling. The shotgun blasts would have pushed the bodies of the victims, in this case those of José and Kitty Menendez, here and there as well. I went on to say that there was no way that, as a forensic pathologist, I could concur with what FAA was claiming. Shooting victims often die right away, so you can't tell how much movement resulted from one particular shot or another, nor how much bleeding was the result of each blast, and so on.

Lyle and Erik Menendez, as we know, were convicted. The jury recommended life imprisonment rather than the death penalty, so it seemed that they believed the sexual abuse allegations. Again, FAA's Roger McCarthy testified for seven-and-a-half days, and his firm was paid more than $1 million for its analysis. But after the trial, the jurors told the attorneys that they had dismissed McCarthy's testimony in about 20 minutes, based upon my rebuttal testimony.

Casey Anthony

Caylee Anthony was a lovely, three-year-old girl who lived in Orlando, Florida, with her mother, Casey, and her maternal grandparents, George and Cindy Anthony.

On July 15, 2008, Caylee was reported missing in a 9-1-1 call placed by Cindy, who had not seen her granddaughter in more than 30 days. Cindy said that Casey had given a variety of explanations as to Caylee's whereabouts before admitting that she had not seen her daughter herself for weeks. Casey then lied to detectives, telling them that her daughter had been kidnapped by a nanny on June 9, and that she had been trying to find her, but to no avail. In October 2008, Casey Anthony was charged with first-degree murder in the death of little Caylee, and pleaded "not guilty." I was consulted initially by José Baez, the lead attorney on the case. But after reviewing the available information, I had come to believe that Casey Anthony was more than likely guilty in the death of her child. Given this, the defense had no use for me.

One problem with the Casey Anthony case was that the prosecution went for first-degree murder. I don't think the jury liked the idea of sending such a young woman, if proven guilty, to jail for the rest of her life. If the prosecution had settled for second-degree murder or manslaughter, I believe they would have gotten a conviction, instead of a widely reviled acquittal.

José Baez strutted in the courtroom like an unctuous trial attorney straight out of a B-movie, and Florida's lead prosecutor, Jeff Ashton, was complacent and extremely harsh in his demeanor. Remember, in most high-profile cases, attorneys on both sides go for drama, and the Casey Anthony trial was no exception. None of this surprised me, given that the trial was televised.

A defendant who is charged with killing a small child starts off with a lot of prejudice against him or her, whereas in a case that involves the murder of an adult, the defense can bring out something negative about the decedent; a scenario that led to their death, such as lies, infidelity, or whatever. But what negative information could you bring out about a small child? Did little Caylee cry too much, or piss her pants too often? Is that what drove whoever to murder her?

From testimony, the jury learned that someone had Googled the word "chloroform" on the Anthony family's computer. A witness described that the air in the trunk of Casey's car smelled of human decomposition. Blow flies were present. The trunk also contained a hair from Caylee's head. When Caylee's remains were discovered, duct tape was found wrapped around her face. Couple all of this with the fact that Casey had failed to report Caylee missing for weeks, and had been lying, non-stop, to her parents and law enforcement. One has to wonder, at what point does the jury's doubt begin to diminish? And at what point does the "reasonableness" of that doubt begin to diminish, too?

It's true that accidents happen, and children sometimes die because of the stupidity, negligence, or inattentiveness of their parents. But I believe that the jury in the Casey Anthony case simply could not fathom why an attractive young mother, if she wanted her freedom, would have elected to kill her daughter rather than just leaving her in the care of her parents. And if Caylee had actually drowned, as was mysteriously alleged by the defense at trial, odds are that the case would have been written off as just a tragic accident. The most that would have happened, even with an aggressive prosecuting attorney, would have been a charge of involuntary manslaughter, for which someone with a clean record would get probation, or maybe a year or two in jail.

Casey Anthony languished in jail for three years awaiting trial and never said a word about Caylee drowning. Then her defense alleged that Casey's father, a former law-enforcement officer, after this "tragic accident" supposedly occurred, decided to discard his beloved grandchild in a swamp not far from his home. If I had been sitting on that jury, I would have considered Casey Anthony the lowest form of human being imaginable; totally narcissistic and amazingly stupid. Who would sit in jail for three years facing a murder charge and run the risk of being sentenced to life in prison if their child truly had drowned by accident? What about Casey's father, George Anthony? Why wouldn't he have come forward and said something? What the hell was that jury thinking?

The Casey Anthony trial presented many conundrums for American jurisprudence, including to what degree did the so-called "CSI Effect" determine the outcome. Jurors for the case were perplexed by the fact that the prosecution couldn't tell them with any certainty when, where and how little Caylee Anthony died. Today, the general American public, as viewers of CSI-based media programs, tend to go looking for the kinds of things that they have seen portrayed on TV. I'm not saying that this was the sole or principal factor in the debacle that was the Casey Anthony trial and verdict, but I would bet anything that it was a factor, based upon some of the questions that jurors asked in the media afterward.

"Why was Casey's DNA not found on the duct tape that encircled Caylee's face?" Because six months in a swamp, coupled with the natural decomposition process, would have destroyed any traces of the perpetrator's DNA. That jury was looking for

DNA, and they didn't get it. They needed a "smoking gun" to convict. And, as any trial lawyer knows, such a thing seldom appears.

Chandra Levy

In May of 2001, Chandra Levy, an intern at the Federal Bureau of Prisons in Washington, D.C., went missing. At the time, the media had run wild with stories of the young woman's alleged affair with California Congressman Gary Condit. But Condit had a convincing alibi for the time when Chandra disappeared: He was in meetings with the Vice President of the United States. As a result, Gary Condit was never named a suspect by police and was eventually cleared of any involvement in Chandra Levy's disappearance. Sadly, the attention that had been focused on Ms. Levy's connection to Mr. Condit wasted time that should have been spent searching for her. (Gary Condit was defeated in his re-election bid the next year.)

Henry Lee, Michael Baden and I were called down to D.C. to check things out. In my opinion, after Chandra's disappearance, the local police conducted neither a thorough investigation nor a thorough search for her. If a proper search had been done, the authorities likely would have found her body, and would then have had evidence that I believe would have led to her killer.

A year after her disappearance, almost to the day, Chandra Levy's remains were discovered in Rock Creek Park, but all that was left of her were her bones. There was no DNA and, therefore, there was nothing we could do to help solve the case, really.

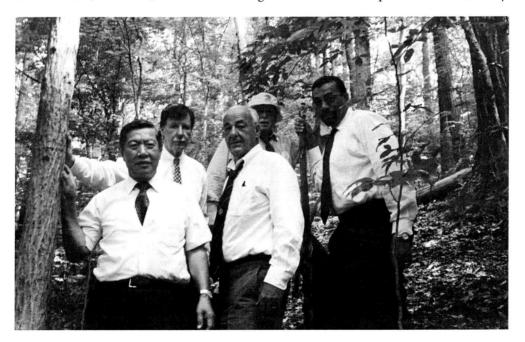

Levy family attorney Billy Martin (far right) brings Dr. Henry Lee, investigator Joseph McCann (back left), me, and Dr. Michael Baden (back center) to the site where Chandra Levy's remains were found, 2002 (Dr. Henry Lee).

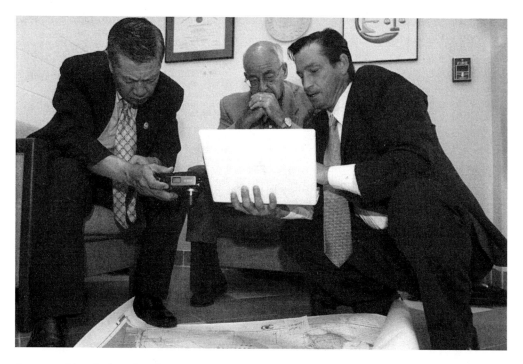

Attorney Matt Dalton briefs Dr. Henry Lee and me on the Scott Peterson case, 2002 (Polaris Images/Debbie Noda).

Nevertheless, Michael Baden, Henry Lee and I examined Chandra Levy's bones at the D.C. Medical Examiner's Office, and we identified a defect in the hyoid bone which suggested that Chandra's death was due to manual strangulation. But in my mind, there was a question as to whether or not the man who was eventually arrested and charged with her murder was the true killer.

Ingmar Guandique, an illegal immigrant from El Salvador, had been known to haunt the Rock Creek Park area in search of young women. He was convicted of murdering Chandra Levy in November 2010, and sentenced to 60 years in prison, but was ultimately granted a new trial after a successful appeal. In July 2016, prosecutors decided that they would not proceed with the case against Ingmar Guandique. Eight months later, he lost his bid to remain in the U.S. and was deported to his native El Salvador.

Kurt Cobain

I addressed the death of rock star Kurt Cobain back when it occurred in 1994, and that's how filmmakers Ben Statler and Donnie Eichar came to contact me. From a forensic science standpoint, I find it strange that a person would inject themselves with heroin, withdraw the needle, detach it and the tourniquet, put everything back into a nice, little drug paraphernalia kit, and then pick up a shotgun and shoot himself.

BEN STATLER: *Dr. Wecht saved the day in a number of ways with our film* Soaked in Bleach, *by just being who he is, with his solid reputation. And Tom Grant [the private investigator who has never let go of the case because he believes that Kurt Cobain was murdered] was thrilled to have Dr. Wecht come on board for the project, to back up what he's always said.*

As I understood it, the film was intended to examine the Kurt Cobain case to show that the "facts," as established by the Seattle authorities, didn't make sense and, as a result, the case should be reopened. Truth and justice were the goals.

DONNIE EICHAR: *I did a lot of research trying to find a forensic scientist and, in my opinion, there's no one better to separate fact from fiction in the Kurt Cobain case than Dr. Wecht. He has studied some of the most well-known death cases in modern history, and seemed like a real straight-shooter. That's what we needed in reviewing the case.*

I broke the Kurt Cobain case down into three parts. First, science did not support a suicide by gunshot because the amount of heroin in Cobain's system was extremely high, which would have rendered him unable to handle a shotgun. Second, investigators never interviewed people related to the case. And third, within a few hours, the Seattle authorities had labeled the death a suicide, which was totally premature. They botched the case, and haven't released a lot of things, such as crime-scene photos and certain autopsy documents, which is infuriating.

DONNIE EICHAR: *What amazed me was Dr. Wecht's attention to the smallest of details. He was discovering things that investigators, for the last 20 years, hadn't found just by reviewing the data, the records and the police reports.*

I was pleased because both Ben and Donnie were pleased. They felt that I did a good job, so good, in fact, that they wanted more and came to Pittsburgh for a second filming of two or three hours.

DONNIE EICHAR: *When I went to interview him, Dr. Wecht was all business. He shook my hand, and said, jokingly, "Where's hair and makeup? Let's get on with this." He was such a professional and so eloquent in the way he spoke, and I was blown away when he started talking about comparable cases. His memory is encyclopedic. And he's a natural on camera. He lures you in with his charm. He doesn't lead on that he has any special interest in a case, and then explodes with information at the right time. It was amazing to see how passionate he is. Dr. Wecht is whip-smart. I just wanted the cream of the crop, the "godfather of forensic pathology." I actually didn't think I would be able to get him for our film. It's not like he needs another credit or more press coverage. But he took the time to be a part of it for no other reason than he believes that the investigation had been botched and the truth needed to be told. In a way, he's a voice for voiceless victims.*

BEN STATLER: *Before* Soaked in Bleach, *it was always possible to marginalize Tom Grant as just another private investigator. But since we had Dr. Wecht reinforcing the points Tom had been making about the toxicology and other elements of the investigation, people couldn't ignore the case anymore.*

Jeffrey Epstein

On July 6, 2019, Jeffrey Epstein, a 66-year-old, wealthy financier, was arrested at Teterboro Airport in New Jersey on federal charges of conspiracy in sex-trafficking dozens of underage girls in Florida and New York. Epstein was a convicted sex offender who was given a "sweetheart" plea deal back in 2008, and served only 13 months of confinement, with work-release privileges.

Having been denied bail this time around, Epstein was remanded to the Metropolitan Correctional Center (MCC) in Manhattan where, on July 23, after one (questionable) attempt to take his own life, he was placed on "suicide watch." Six days later, inexplicably, Epstein was removed from said watch list, with the proviso that he be checked by guards every 30 minutes. But that procedure was not followed on the night of August 9, when over-worked and slumbering guards had left Epstein alone for several hours.

On the morning of August 10, Jeffrey Epstein was discovered hanging in his jail cell, and was pronounced dead from cardiac arrest after being taken to a local hospital. So, did Jeffrey Epstein commit suicide, or was he a victim of foul play? The initial ruling of the Chief Medical Examiner of New York City, Dr. Barbara Sampson, was designated as "pending." A week later, she announced her final ruling: Jeffrey Epstein had indeed hanged himself and, thus, committed suicide. But I have many questions about this ruling, and the speed in which Dr. Sampson issued it. How could she have made such a definitive ruling so quickly when so much investigative information was yet to be received? Did Dr. Sampson have a clear and total picture of the situation surrounding Jeffrey Epstein's death?

The autopsy of Jeffrey Epstein showed that he had suffered a fracture of the hyoid bone and the thyroid cartilage: the "Adam's Apple." Cervical breaks are common in hanging deaths. And breaks in the thyroid cartilage can be detected, on occasion, in the bodies of people who have hanged themselves, especially if they were older. However, for a hanging to break the thyroid cartilage and the hyoid bone, the amount of force on the drop would have had to be substantial, and the drop for Jeffrey Epstein could not have been higher than the top bunk in his cell. A broken hyoid bone is much more common in people who have been strangled. Barbara Sampson, a solid professional, knows this, and studies exist that support it.

MICHAEL BADEN: *I was there for the autopsy, on behalf of the Epstein family and Mr. Epstein's estate. Soon after, I discussed the case with Cyril, and he and I both agreed that three fractures in the neck is indicative of homicide, not suicide. But one must have access to all the pertinent information to be able to make a final decision, such as the position of Epstein's body at the time he was found; what the other inmates saw or heard; and what the lab results were. Such information is available, but the U.S. Department of Justice says they can't release it because trials for two indicted prison guards have not yet occurred.*

In any case, here's some of what Dr. Sampson may not have considered at the time of her ruling. No matter how understaffed the MCC was, it was inexcusable for a high-profile defendant such as Jeffrey Epstein to be left unattended long enough for him to kill himself (if that is what happened). It is not easy for an inmate to die by suicide in a jail cell when he or she is watched properly. Mafia crime boss John Gotti, investment swindler Bernard Madoff, and the Mexican drug lord "El Chapo" had all been housed at the MCC, and lived to be tried and convicted. If the authorities are careful with regard to the make-up of the clothing and bedding provided to the in-mate, thus making certain that nothing could be used as a makeshift ligature, suicide is no longer a viable method to escape justice. Where were Epstein's guards on the night of August 9? And why did several of them "lawyer-up" and refuse to cooperate with the investigation?

It is reportedly standard practice at the MCC for inmates on suicide watch to be assigned a cellmate, a person to provide company for an inmate with suicidal tenden-cies, who could alert guards in the event that an emergency arises. In the case of Jeffrey Epstein, his last cellmate was transferred out of the MCC's Special Housing Unit just hours before Epstein's death. Why did the MCC break protocol and leave Epstein alone in his cell? And, in the portion of the housing unit in which Jeffrey Epstein was being held, why were the surveillance cameras not working in the hours preceding, during and after his death?

Given who Jeffrey Epstein was, what he had allegedly done, and the prominence of the people who were connected with him, his death remains a highly suspicious case. Had he lived, we likely would have unearthed, during his trial, a "Pandora's Box" of lurid goings-on and the names of some famous and powerful people who delighted in the same things that Jeffrey Epstein did.

Maybe Jeffrey Epstein did commit suicide, but I'm not so sure about that. A person can be suffocated or strangled, and then posed for a hanging. I've had a few cases like that over the years. Given all of the investigations that are still being conducted con-cerning Epstein's death, and those that may be opened in the future, my finding would have remained "pending." I said as much in interviews with some newspapers, on CNN, on Fox News with Dana Perino, and live on Fox with Judge Jeanine Pirro.

◆ ◆ ◆

You have now been briefed on my involvement in and/or opinions about some of the most high-profile cases in recent U.S. history. Let's look back in time at some other fascinating cases, some of which you will know; others may have been lost to your memory due to the passage of time.

Elvis Presley

Elvis Presley, the greatest American cultural icon of his or, perhaps, any era, and the best-selling music artist worldwide, was a relatively young man, in his early 40s, when he was found unconscious, suddenly and unexpectedly, on August 16, 1977, at Graceland, his home in Memphis, Tennessee.

Around 2:30 p.m., Elvis' girlfriend, Ginger Alden, discovered the music star lying face down on the floor of his bathroom, and called for help. Within minutes, an ambu-lance arrived to transport the all-but-lifeless singer to Methodist South Hospital, which was located just five minutes from Graceland. It was then that Elvis's personal physician, Dr. George Nichopoulos, ordered the driver to take Elvis to Baptist Memorial Hospital instead, which was 21 minutes away, believing that the staff there would be more discreet about the matter. At Baptist Memorial, life-saving efforts were undertaken, but to no avail, and Elvis Presley was pronounced dead at 3:30 p.m.

On that same day, Dr. Jerry Francisco, the local Chief Medical Examiner, took command. Even though Dr. Francisco said that he didn't believe that Presley's death was a medical examiner's case, Elvis' family insisted on an autopsy, and one was performed at Baptist Memorial by a respected pathologist named Dr. E. Eric Muirhead. But long before microscopic tissues had been examined and before toxicological analyses had been completed, Jerry Francisco, at 8 p.m., on August 16, announced that Elvis had died from cardiac arrest due to heart disease. It was he who also stated that drugs played no role in the singer's death. Dr. Francisco's statement was not only premature; it was the wrong thing to do.

Soon thereafter, I got a call from ABC's "20/20" news magazine. They had obtained Elvis' autopsy report and asked me if I would give them my opinion about what it said. They sent it to me and I reviewed it. Sure, Elvis' heart was a little enlarged. (He was a very big guy at that time.) But based upon what was contained in the report, I determined that Elvis Presley had not died from heart disease, but rather from drug toxicity. So, they came and interviewed me, and I explained.

I knew Jerry Francisco from the American Academy of Forensic Sciences, and he was an arrogant S.O.B. I never discussed the Presley autopsy with him because, among all of my colleagues, nobody disputed my take on things. In essence, Elvis Presley was the victim of polypharmacy (the same condition that rendered Sunny von Bülow comatose), and I made this case repeatedly on news programs at the time. Elvis' doctor or doctors provided him with many drugs. When Elvis died, he had 12 central nervous system depressant drugs in his system, the combination of which led to his death. And one side-effect of those drugs is constipation. The poor man spent three or four hours a day in the bathroom toward the end of his otherwise magnificent life.

Elvis Presley was a major industry in America. I remember reading once that one out of every 12 people in America owned at least one of his records. "The King" meant big business for Tennessee, and if it got out that he died from drug abuse, that might blacken, besmirch, or diminish the attractiveness of his celebrity. Perhaps some government or business people put pressure on Jerry Francisco to get ahead of the story. I don't know. But I believe that was probably true. There must be an answer to why he did what he did. Toxicology results would have come back to him in a couple of days, and there was no way that they would remain a secret, not when they pertained to the death of one of the most famous people in world.

Jean Harris

Jean Harris was the headmistress of the Madeira School for Girls in McLean, Virginia. She made national news in the early 1980s when she was tried and convicted of shooting and killing her ex-lover, Dr. Herman Tarnower, a well-known cardiologist and author of the best-selling book, *The Complete Scarsdale Medical Diet*.

A criminalist/ballistics consultant and I spoke with Jean Harris and she described a struggle with Dr. Tarnower over the gun used in the incident, in clear and specific detail. I really believed her story. She went to see her boyfriend, Dr. Tarnower, from whom she was then estranged, and was so distraught about their breakup that she intended to kill herself. Tarnower was having an affair with a young nurse and, when confronted by Jean with a gun in her hand, he struggled to gain control, and the gun went off several times, after which Herman Tarnower collapsed and died.

The case was a great disappointment for me. I believe that Jean Harris could have prevailed in court by playing to the sympathy of the jury, but she came across as arrogant. While giving testimony, she shed not a tear and expressed not a moment of regret or remorse, so the jurors expressed themselves by declaring her "guilty."

Defense attorneys must prepare their clients to perform well on the stand. Defendants must be advised about how to dress, how to walk, how to talk, how to sit, when to look at the jury, and when not to look. It is possible that Jean Harris' lawyers did their best to prepare her for testifying, but perhaps she was too stubborn to heed their advice. After all, she was a very proud woman.

Charles Manson

The Manson Family was a cult formed in California in the late 1960s. Led by Charles Manson, a wily and intelligent ex-con, the group consisted of roughly 100 followers who lived an unconventional lifestyle that included free and open sexuality, and the habitual use of hallucinogenic drugs. Anyone who was conscious in the summer of 1969 can remember the shocking murders committed by several of Manson's loyal followers at the behest of their leader.

On the night of August 8, 1969, Manson directed several members of his "family" to go to a specific address and kill everyone present. They did, but they made a mess of things. The next night, Manson accompanied a similar group to another home, intending to show them how to do it right. Again, the followers did what Manson had asked and murdered the occupants of the house, but Manson, cleverly and for his own preservation, had left before the killing started.

I was a consultant to my friend, Dr. Tom Noguchi, who was then the Medical Examiner of Los Angeles County, and I reviewed the case for him. I was not involved in the trial, but I thought that Charles Manson and his cohorts were all guilty of murder and, in time, the jury saw it that way.

Tom Noguchi: *Many high-profile people live in the Los Angeles area, and Hollywood has a continuing idea that everything that happens there should be kept secret. But some people die in conditions in which a medical examiner must launch an official investigation. Once you do it, you cannot hide from the fact that you are required to say what happened, and you can't please everyone. I learned from Cyril that the only way to handle things is to walk a straight line, knowing that some people will be unhappy. Like Cyril, I would rather be respected than liked.*

Later on, I came to know Vincent Bugliosi, the Manson case prosecutor, when legendary attorney Jerry Spence and I took part with Vince in a mock trial of Lee Harvey Oswald for the assassination of JFK, which was filmed in London. Vince and I started off as serious antagonists but, over the years, we developed a healthy respect and friendship.

I corresponded with Bugliosi for years and his family even asked me to deliver a eulogy at his funeral in 2015. (Unfortunately, I couldn't do it because I wasn't available on the date.) In his book about the JFK assassination, *Reclaiming History*, in which Bugliosi defends the Warren Commission Report, there is a chapter in which he talks favorably about me and considers me to be the most serious, knowledgeable, intelligent and objective of the Warren Commission's critics.

Chappaquiddick

On July 18, 1969, U.S. Senator Ted Kennedy was driving home from a party with a young woman when his car plunged off a narrow bridge into a saltwater pond on Chappaquiddick Island in Massachusetts. Teddy survived, but his passenger, 28-year-old Mary Jo Kopechne, didn't. I believe, almost certainly, that she drowned.

Senator Kennedy could have been charged with involuntary manslaughter, especially since he left the scene after the accident. In that sense, I don't think justice was served. But I also don't think that there was any evidence of foul play of a deliberate nature. It's too bad that Mary Jo's body wasn't exhumed just to establish, unequivocally, that her death was due to drowning, and that there was nothing else to it. Incredibly, no autopsy was ever done.

F. LEE BAILEY: *On Chappaquiddick, if a forensic pathologist came up with something that wasn't helpful to law enforcement, they'd hold it against him. A lot of forensic pathologists work day-in and day-out with the cops and, although they may not lie for them, they don't want to embarrass them for fear of getting punished. I thought that Cyril, who couldn't be intimidated if you faced him with a Sherman tank, would have been ideal for this case because he had the right credentials, a lot of credibility, and is an outstanding witness.*

Edmund Dinis, the DA of Suffolk County was, initially, being criticized for picking on Teddy Kennedy. Then when he made it known that he wasn't going to prosecute, he was threatened with impeachment because many said that the case had been "fixed."

Years later, Ed Dinis contacted Lee Bailey seeking a forensic pathology expert. Lee recommended me, so Dinis called and asked if I would review the Kopechne case and testify before a judge in Luzerne County in order to obtain permission for the exhumation and autopsy of Mary Jo's body. So, I reviewed everything and we met and talked. Then I went to Luzerne County and testified.

At the end of the day, the judge was very complimentary and expressed his beliefs that an autopsy should have been done immediately after Mary Jo died. However, in light of the Kopechne family's adamant objections to the exhumation, and in light of the fact that no formal legal action had been initiated by the DA—such as a charge of "vehicular homicide" or "involuntary manslaughter" against Ted Kennedy—he did not have the basis to grant Ed's wishes. I don't mean to criticize Ed Dinis, because he had endured great pressure from all sides on this case. But if he had filed a formal legal action of some sort, which he wouldn't have been obligated to see through, it would have been all the judge needed to grant our request.

Why was the Kopechne family so adamant about not having an autopsy? My belief is that they, as devout Roman Catholics, were concerned about us getting into questions about Mary Jo's sexual history and lifestyle. Considering their background, these were not irrational concerns. I can understand their position. Their daughter was dead and they just preferred to let it be. Where would such an investigation lead, anyway? Ted Kennedy was responsible for Mary Jo's death. And I'm not suggesting that anything improper took place on the part of Teddy Kennedy and his insurance company, but had the Kopechnes received any remuneration for their loss? I don't know.

The role of the family's religious beliefs, in time, was confirmed. A couple of decades later, I was invited to speak at a Luzerne County Bar Association meeting for a post-graduate program in forensic science. When I was finished, an elderly man approached me and introduced himself, and we chatted. He told me that he had been the Kopechne's attorney at the time of the tragedy at Chappaquiddick. He also told me that the family's reason for objecting to the autopsy was their concern about the very things I mentioned regarding sexual activity, and so on.

About a year or two ago, Mrs. Kopechne was interviewed, for whatever reason, and she said, in tears, that the thing she regretted most in her life was objecting to the initial autopsy. She still had questions about what had happened. I think it's straightforward that Ted Kennedy was likely drunk and was driving, in a hurry, to a place where he and Mary Jo could have sex. The entrance to the bridge curves and the bridge itself is narrow, and he lost control of his car. That's horrible as it is. But what is more horrible is Teddy's leaving the scene of the accident and going back to his motel. That was a crime.

Jeffrey MacDonald

Jeffrey MacDonald was a United States Army officer and board-certified emergency room physician, whom everybody seemed to like and respect. He had a beautiful wife and two adorable daughters, ages 2 and 5. In the wee hours of February 17, 1970, MacDonald's wife, Colette, and his two little girls were brutally murdered in their home on the Fort Bragg military base in North Carolina. Jeffrey, who was discovered with a single stab wound in his chest, said that intruders had entered his home and yelled things such as "kill the pigs." The next thing he knew, he woke up and found his family dead. The authorities didn't believe him, so Jeffrey MacDonald was charged with murder.

When the case came before a military tribunal, MacDonald was acquitted, and the stepfather of his deceased wife, Freddie Kassab, along with Jeffrey's mother-in-law, were in his corner. But they turned on him when Jeffrey moved from North Carolina to California to make a fresh start, and began to date. The parents felt that he was betraying their daughter by not remaining loyal to his wife's memory. So, Kassab became MacDonald's nemesis, and continued to pursue the case with a passionate desire that was not susceptible to any kind of reasoning. Ultimately, Kassab succeeded. The case was reopened and, this time, it would be heard in a civilian court.

I was consulted and went to testify in the case, but wound up not doing so after the judge ruled that, since another forensic pathologist had already testified, my testimony would have been little more than repetition. But I remember being there and, of course, working with the defense attorneys. And I do not believe that the evidence was sufficient to convict Jeffrey MacDonald.

For one thing, the military authorities at Fort Bragg had failed to investigate thoroughly the daughter of one of the colonels at the base who was part of a group of young people who cavorted about late at night dressed in witch's garb. This was in the days of Charles Manson and his murderous "family," so the idea that such a group of young miscreants could have perpetrated the crime that took place at the MacDonald home was not far-fetched. At one point, one member of the group confessed, saying that he had been involved in the murders of Jeffrey MacDonald's wife and children. But later on, he recanted, and the possibility of the colonel's daughter's involvement was never pursued further.

To think that Jeffrey MacDonald committed this crime is hard for me to believe. He had no motive, and I think that, by no means, could the ultimate "guilty" verdict have been sustained "beyond a reasonable doubt." But why did Jeffrey MacDonald end up with but a single stab wound when his wife and kids were murdered with such fury? It's a good question that does create some doubt as to the veracity of Jeffrey's story. On the other hand, once MacDonald was incapacitated, a group of young people, perhaps hopped-up on hallucinogenic drugs and under the influence of witchcraft, could have committed the crime.

F. LEE BAILEY: *In my view, Jeffrey MacDonald, in fact, saw his house invaded. He had no motive whatever to kill his wife and children, but he got scared and hid in a closet, and couldn't afford, as long as he lived, to tell anybody. His survival instinct probably took over and he avoided getting killed himself. Even though he was a doctor and not a combatant, MacDonald wore a military uniform. For a military man, that kind of cowardice is probably a worse condemnation than if he had killed his family. You just can't stand by and watch that happen. If he did, it's a story he can never, ever tell, and he certainly never has.*

Jeffrey MacDonald remains one of the most puzzling cases of all for me. From a strictly legal standpoint, I don't think the prosecution proved their case. They had no strong evidence. But am I totally comfortable with the notion that Jeffrey did not commit those murders?

I want to make it clear: Legally, I don't believe that the prosecution proved his guilt, but MacDonald's was a case from which the jury couldn't walk away, especially in those days. A woman and two children were not just murdered; they were slaughtered. And there wasn't an alternative defendant to consider. I'm not sure of what happened. I can't say that I can prove that Jeffrey is innocent, although I've expressed that many times. But the verdict that was handed down in this case is one of which I am not quite certain.

Jeffrey MacDonald was convicted of murder and sent to prison for life. I have not corresponded with him, recently, but I had done so, for period of years, a number of times. I sent him books, as a matter of personal courtesy. And I have corresponded with his second wife, who has worked vigorously for many years trying to have Jeffrey's conviction overturned. There's nothing inappropriate about these actions on my part, as long as I never sent a hacksaw hidden in a birthday cake.

◆ ◆ ◆

I don't want you to get the idea that I'm only interested in famous, media-driven cases, with luminary defendants or victims. As I've said, I get involved in cases of all types, for all kinds of reasons. Some are riveting. Some are strange. And some are downright frustrating. What follows are summations of some cases from my past that are not as well known. They might surprise you.

Delbert Ward

I felt good about the case of Delbert Ward, probably more so than any other case in which I'd been involved. I heard about it, contacted the defense attorney, and he brought me on board.

In a rural farming community called Munnsville, near Utica, New York, the four elderly and barely literate Ward brothers—William, Roscoe, Lyman and Delbert—lived together on a small family farm after their parents died, in a tarpaper shack with no running water and no electricity. One morning, in 1990, William Ward, who had been ill for years, was found dead, and brother Delbert was accused of murdering him, perhaps by suffocation, as an act of mercy. But did Delbert Ward have a motive or even the capacity to kill his brother?

Maddening as it was, this case was also heartwarming. The townsfolk came together and held bake sales and so forth to raise a few dollars to support Delbert in his time of need. It was astounding to see the remaining brothers enter the courtroom in suits that maybe they had worn only once, when their parents died.

I worked on the case *pro bono*, and learned quickly that the local medical examiner had made many errors. He was one of those medical examiners who listens to what the prosecution wants, and gives it to them. On the stand, I took his findings apart, point-by-point, until there was nothing left of them. Thanks to my testimony, and hard work by his attorney, Delbert Ward was acquitted.

So, I've been involved in many cases where I've testified for the prosecution and people have been found "guilty" and others in which my testimony has led to acquittals. It works both ways.

A final note on the Delbert Ward case: Filmmakers Joe Berlinger and Bruce Sinofsky produced an insightful documentary about the case called *Brother's Keeper*, which won the Audience Award for Documentary at the Sundance Film Festival in 1992, among other honors. I am depicted as I testified in court.

Legionnaires' Disease

On July 21, 1976, the American Legion opened its statewide convention at the Bellevue-Stratford Hotel in Philadelphia. More than 2,000 "Legionnaires" attended, most of whom were men. Three days after the convention concluded, on July 27, Legionnaire Ray Brennan, a 61-year-old retired U.S. Air Force Captain and a bookkeeper for the American Legion, died at his home of an apparent heart attack. He had returned home from the convention on the evening of July 24 complaining of feeling tired.

On July 30, another Legionnaire, Frank Aveni, age 60, also died of an apparent heart attack, as did three other Legionnaires, all of whom had been convention attendees. By August 1, six more Legionnaires had died, all having complained of tiredness, chest pains, lung congestion and fever. Within a week, more than 130 people, mostly men, had been hospitalized, and 25 had died.

The Legionnaire's case was less of a "who-dunit" than a "what-dunit." Fortunately, the U.S. Centers for Disease Control (CDC) and the Pennsylvania Health Department responded quickly. I spoke out about the situation and gained lots of media coverage about this serious issue on TV, and even in the *New York Times*. In November 1976, I testified before the U.S. House Subcommittee on Consumer Protection, and was also appointed to a national committee to review the case.

In 1977, Dr. Joseph McDade of the CDC discovered a new bacterium that was identified as the causative organism of the disease that had sickened and killed so many. It thrives in hot, damp places, such as the water of the cooling towers for the Bellevue-Stratford's air-conditioning system, which spread the disease throughout the hotel. The bacterium was named "legionella," and the disease "legionellosis," after the first victims.

In the end, 149 Legionnaires had become ill, as well as 33 others who were associated with the hotel, or were in the area at the time of the convention. Of these 182 cases, 29 people had died.

The negative publicity associated with the outbreak (in which I played a major role) caused occupancy at the Bellevue-Stratford to plummet to just four percent, and the hotel finally closed on November 18, 1976.

Alien Autopsy

I was thinking about the television program "Alien Autopsy: Truth or Fiction?" and wasn't sure about whether or not I should include it in this book. But I decided that, while it was not an important case, I'd like to explain my participation in it.

In 1995, I got a call from Fox television to join some well-known people to view a 17-minute black-and-white film depicting a secret medical examination and autopsy of a purported extra-terrestrial being, or "alien," by the U.S. military.

After seeing the film, I was asked, on camera, for my impressions, to which I replied, "The autopsy procedures featured appear authentic." I also said that, and these were my exact words, "It looked like no body that I had ever seen." I never said that the autopsy subject was actually an alien. I said that further examinations would have to be done.

I didn't conduct this "alien autopsy," but it was interesting to see the film, and I wasn't paid anything. I got to meet and speak with Oscar-winning special-effects make-up artist Stan Winston, cinematographer Allen Daviau, and Kevin Randle, a noted UFO author and investigator. Not one of us believed that the film was authentic. It turned out, in the end, that the whole thing was a fraud perpetrated by a man named Ray Santilli.

I don't want to say that I don't believe in the possibility of extraterrestrial beings, because I have no knowledge of what's out there. There are trillions of stars and planets, and I think it is intellectually arrogant for people to say that we're the only sophisticated lifeform in our solar system. I have an open mind, and it was with that spirit that I approached the project.

Kenneth Minor

The Kenneth Minor case was a strange one. In New York City, a motivational speaker and self-help author named Jeffrey Locker approached a man named Kenneth Minor for help in staging Locker's actual death, in what would look like a knifing and robbery. Why? So that Locker's family could collect on his life insurance.

Jeffrey Minor complied, and stabbed Locker to death on an East Harlem street in Locker's automobile. But in the U.S., "assisted suicide" always was and still is, illegal. Initially, the detectives and the district attorney understandably believed that this was a "homicide." However, after interviewing Locker's wife and reviewing all of the background information, they reluctantly came to realize that Minor's story was true.

Prosecutors admitted that Locker had asked Minor to help him stage his death, but said that Minor went beyond assisted suicide when he stabbed Locker a total of seven times. So, rather than charging Minor with manslaughter, the prosecutors pushed for second-degree murder, even though it was recognized and accepted that Minor had been solicited to do the killing.

I reenacted the stabbing in the courtroom, and then in a garage across the street, for television. This happened in 2009 and, in 2011, Kenneth Minor, the "Harlem Kevorkian," was convicted of murder and sentenced to 20-years-to-life in prison. His conviction was later overturned on appeal, and Minor accepted a plea deal that reduced his 20-year sentence to 12 years.

The case of Kenneth Minor was a disappointment. Even with his sentence reduction, the deal still carried a conviction for murder rather than a reduction of the crime to manslaughter, which I think was unfair.

Dr. Robert Ferrante

On April 17, 2013, Dr. Amber Klein, a neurologist, left work at UPMC Presbyterian hospital in Pittsburgh around 11 p.m., and made the short walk to her home on Lytton

Avenue, in the Schenley Farms area of Oakland. No more than 30 minutes later, her husband, Dr. Robert Ferrante, a neuro-researcher, discovered her on the floor of their kitchen, struggling to breathe. She died three days later, after being in a deep coma and on life-support.

On April 20, not long after his wife had died, Dr. Ferrante insisted that Amber Klein's body be cremated. But given the unusual nature of her death, blood and tissue samples had already been taken. The Allegheny County Medical Examiner, based on several toxicological reports on Dr. Klein's blood—one from the county lab and another from Quest Diagnostics—determined that she had died from cyanide poisoning. The forensic pathologist then ruled Dr. Klein's death a "homicide," which resulted in Dr. Ferrante being arrested and charged with murder. I was aware that cyanide is found naturally not only in human blood, but in human tissues. Tissue specimens of Amber Klein were available, but no further testing was conducted.

The Allegheny County Medical Examiner's Office used what is called a "diffusion color test" to determine simply if cyanide was present in Amber Klein's blood. The indicator turned purple, so cyanide was considered to be present. Quest Diagnostics first reported the cyanide level in Dr. Klein's blood at 3.4 milligrams/liter, which they subsequently corrected to 2.2 mg/L. So, right there, you have a question about whether or not Quest knew what it was doing. If I were a medical examiner, faced with conflicting toxicological numbers, I would stop everything and initiate further testing in another lab before determining a cause of death. But the prosecution never bothered to resolve the conflict. They simply ran with Quest's test findings.

There's a company in Willow Grove, Pennsylvania, called National Medical Services (NMS), which is considered to be the premier forensic toxicology lab in the U.S. Name the case where drugs have been an issue, and they have either done the original testing or the follow-up tests for corroboration and validation. NMS's first test of Amber Klein's blood, which was initiated by the defense, was deemed "inconclusive." But on a second run-through, it came in with a normal cyanide level of 0.3 to 0.5 mg/L.

At Dr. Ferrante's trial, Bill Difenderfer, the lead defense counsel, chose to put three forensic science experts on the stand. Dr. Robert Middleberg, from NMS, said that tests on Amber Klein's blood at his facility were inconclusive, and his testimony was supported by both Dr. Shaun Carstairs of the Naval Medical Center in San Diego, California, and me.

When I finished my testimony, I exited the courtroom and was greeted by a crowd of reporters. NBC's "Dateline," CBS's "48 Hours," and lots of other media were present. A phrase that was tossed around by several reporters was, "Dr. Wecht, your testimony was a game-changer." When they bumped into each other after the Ferrante trial, an Allegheny County judge told my son-in-law that Jeffrey Manning—the judge in the Ferrante case—said that, after my testimony, he thought the defense probably was going to win an acquittal. Bill Difenderfer and Wendy Williams, the defense attorneys, and I all felt that, at the very least, we would get a hung jury. I was in Los Angeles when I heard that the jury had handed down a verdict of "guilty," and was stunned.

It's interesting to note that the Center for Organ Recovery and Education (CORE) harvested Dr. Klein's liver and kidneys and allowed them to be implanted in three patients who were in need of them. Why would they do this if the prosecution was correct about the decedent's cyanide level?

If you believe the test results from the prosecution's side, the cells of Amber Klein's tissues had to have been damaged from such an elevated cyanide level. There's an enzyme called cytochrome oxidase that allows oxygen to be moved from one's arteries to one's cells, and that enzyme is blocked by cyanide. So, even if you have 100 percent oxygen in your arteries, if none of it is getting into your cells, the cells begin to change, and not for the better.

At the Ferrante trial, I testified about the qualifications of NMS, but the prosecution didn't give a damn. "To wrap it up Dr. Wecht, what is your conclusion?" they asked. I said, "The cause of Dr. Amber Klein's death is undetermined and, therefore, the manner of death is undetermined."

Two additional tests were performed by NMS for the principal metabolite thiocyanate, the number-one breakdown product of cyanide, and it was within normal limits. How would the prosecution and their experts explain this? The NMS specimen had not been drawn in a timely manner and wasn't tested for a couple of weeks. So, the prosecution's argument was that, in that time, the level of cyanide had dropped from 2.2, the corrected Quest level, to NMS's 0.3–0.5. Sometimes a cyanide level will drop after death and sometimes it will increase. Nobody knows for sure which way it will go. But if it drops, it doesn't drop from 2.2 to a 0.3–0.5 just because the specimen has been sitting for a couple of weeks.

I also pointed out things that had been ignored by the prosecution. For instance, CORE had a pathologist located in Minnesota who did the exam of Amber Klein's heart. She reported focal fibrosis on three of four heart valves, which means that there had been some insult to the organ. She also reported some dysplastic intramyocardial heart fibers. "Dysplastic" means abnormal. Her findings indicated that Dr. Klein had dysplastic intramyocardial arteries and, hence, there was the distinct possibility of focal disruption of the heart's electrical conduction system. "Focal disruption" means a break in continuity.

CORE's pathologist didn't want to come in from Minnesota for the trial, so I didn't get to see her slides. But we needed to know just how severe the focal disruption was in Amber Klein's heart. I said in my testimony that I could not state with "reasonable medical certainty" that Amber Klein had a cardiac arrhythmia, collapsed and died from that. But I also could not state and did not believe that it could be stated, again with reasonable medical certainty, that she died from cyanide poisoning. In the face of inconsistent and disparate reports from two different laboratories (especially since a finding of a normal cyanide level came from the foremost lab in the country), it is difficult to understand how the jury failed to recognize "reasonable doubt."

The prosecution presented four medical experts and the defense, a like number. One of the jurors, after the trial, was quoted as saying, "The woman from Quest said she'd been doing these tests for 37 years, so we considered her findings valid." That's the way they dealt with the cyanide issue. But this woman was just a lab technician. Forget the testimony of Dr. Middleberg, a board-certified, internationally-recognized forensic toxicologist. Forget also that the Quest technician hails from the lab that reported different levels of 3.4 and then 2.2, a clear mistake. Was the technician's ability challenged? And what is the definition of "beyond a reasonable doubt"? Juries must deal with this in criminal cases, especially those of first-degree murder. If you have the foremost lab in the country giving you a normal cyanide level and CORE doling out the organs of the deceased to needy recipients, does that not constitute a sufficient degree of evidence to prevent you from coming to a verdict of guilty, beyond a reasonable doubt?

Another thing to consider was the fact that Amber Klein was taking large quantities of creatine in hopes of getting pregnant. Creatine metabolizes after ingestion and among the metabolites that it forms is cyanide. Reportedly, Dr. Klein had a "boyfriend" of sorts in Boston, and there are emails to that effect. She was looking for romance outside her marriage, and Dr. Ferrante was suspicious of it.

In one of the emails, she said that she would be traveling to Boston and would stay with this other man. She then sent a follow-up email saying that her husband had decided to join her on the trip, and she was sorry, but she couldn't stay with him after all. Interestingly, her boyfriend's e-response indicates that the romance was one-sided. He said, "Fine. Both of you can stay here."

Was it likely that Dr. Ferrante had poisoned his wife? Yes, I suppose, but that's not the point. Was there evidence that should have prevented the jury from reaching its verdict? That's the issue. If Ferrante didn't "go-a-Googling," looking up cyanide-related information on the Internet, and if he hadn't purchased cyanide for his lab, he probably wouldn't have been in the courtroom at all. But those searches did him in. The other thing that hurt, significantly, was his testimony in court.

Bill Difenderfer is a realist, and I thought he did well in representing his client. The defense made the decision to allow Ferrante to testify on his own behalf. Unfortunately, when he did, he shed no tears and came across as rather cold and stiff. Legally, of course, the defense didn't have to put him on. But in a case like this, Ferrante had to explain himself. He did attempt to explain his actions, bullshit or not, and most of the things he explained were within the realm of possibility.

Many considered the trial of Dr. Robert Ferrante an open-and-shut case, and they all were wrong. I've testified for defendants in homicide cases more than anybody else in my line of work because many medical examiners and forensic pathologists in medical examiners' offices will not do so. They won't even consult with the defense. I testify more for the prosecution because I do so many autopsies for coroners. And it pisses me off when people say that I'm too old to be reliable, but it doesn't surprise me. People have every right to say such things, but all of it is meaningless because they weren't in the courtroom and don't have detailed knowledge of the case; they don't have the necessary medical or legal background; nor do they have a grasp of forensic science. They know only what they have read in the press or seen on TV. I don't say this to be dismissive or arrogant, but this kind of criticism is of no relevance and, therefore, is of no consequence.

Testifying for the defense doesn't bother me in any way because the prosecution has the unfair advantage of unlimited financial resources; the Feds, especially. Whatever is required to win, they will do it. When prosecutors go after a multi-millionaire on Wall Street, people say, "I wish I could afford his defense team." But this happens rarely. It may be big news in the *Wall Street Journal*, and it may even make some other newspapers but, on a percentage basis, that's one in maybe 10,000 cases. What does the "everyday person" get? Often, a public defender, an inexperienced court-appointed attorney, but even that's unfair.

I don't mean to be disrespectful, but many public defenders are fresh out of law school and want to get experience before they become private attorneys. The law says, "You have a right to counsel," but it doesn't say that you have the right to "skilled counsel." Sure, you have a right, but compared to the veteran prosecutors you will be going up against, your counsel will be outgunned. Furthermore, all too often, court-appointed attorneys are denied funding by the trial judge to pay for outside experts.

◆ ◆ ◆

Some court cases are high-profile, but they're not really important to life as most people know it. As far as cases go, in my career, the JFK assassination was the most important. It was a case of international significance. Some of my medical malpractice liability cases were important, too, because, in them, the physicians' reputations were at stake. And many of my civil cases were important because actions taken by individuals or organizations may have left a person or a family destitute, especially if the breadwinner had been lost.

When someone has died or has been seriously injured unnecessarily, I feel good when I can help their families seek financial redress in civil court. I am proud of my "black lung" cases, for example. Those men had worked underground in coal mines for 30 or 40 years and yet, when they got sick or died from pneumoconiosis and chronic obstructive pulmonary disease, their employers tried to claim that their jobs didn't play any role in their deaths. I also feel good about helping with cases in which people have been harmed by faulty products. And of course, I feel good when I've shown that the police have wrongfully caused somebody's injury or death. But not every case is going to be successful. After all, I'm not a magician. Ultimately, I am just a small component of a complex, multi-faceted system.

Run-ins with Police

Tamir Rice

On November 22, 2014, Tamir Rice, a 12-year-old, African American boy, was shot by 26-year-old, white police officer Timothy Loehmann for pointing a pistol—which was called in as "probably fake"—at random people in the Cudell Recreation Center in

Cleveland, Ohio. The officer fired at the boy within seconds after arriving at the scene. Young Tamir Rice died the next day. The boy's pistol was later found to be an Airsoft replica, a gun that shoots pellets which are often plastic or rubber, and the pain inflicted by them is minor. I was not formally consulted in this case, but was called on to testify.

I could probably list 50 or even more incidents similar to that of Tamir Rice, and they are just the tip of the iceberg. Shootings of black suspects by white police officers happen every day in this country, many of which we never hear about. Such incidents always anger me, so I want to tell you about several in which I have been involved personally.

Amadou Diallo

For the case of Amadou Diallo, I was hired by the famous and outstanding attorney Johnnie Cochran. It involved a 23-year-old immigrant from Guinea who was walking up the steps of his home on February 4, 1999, and was shot 41 times by New York City police, and killed. Mr. Diallo went to pull out his wallet to show his ID and the police, as they often do, claimed that they mistook his wallet for a gun, and pumped him full of lead.

I went to the Medical Examiner's Office in New York City, not at the time of the autopsy but subsequently, and reconstructed all the wounds just to corroborate things that were already a matter of record. There was no conflict as to the number of shots or entrance and exit wounds, so I wrote and filed my report. I didn't testify because the matter had already been resolved, in favor of the New York City Police Department, of course. Fortunately, the Diallo family filed a "wrongful death" suit against New York City that was settled for $3 million—small recompense for the life of a young man.

Michael Brown

On August 9, 2014, Michael Brown, an 18-year-old African American male, was walking with his friend, Dorian Johnson, 22, down the middle of a street in the city of Ferguson, Missouri. Around noon, they encountered a police officer, Darren Wilson, who told them to move off the street.

Officer Wilson claimed that, when he told the young men to clear the street, an altercation ensued in which Brown attacked him in his police vehicle in an attempt to get control of Wilson's firearm. But Dorian Johnson stated that Wilson had initiated the confrontation by grabbing Brown by the neck through his car window, threatening and, ultimately, shooting at him, after which Brown and Johnson fled the scene. Wilson then stated that Brown stopped and charged him after a short pursuit, but Johnson contradicted this account as well, stating that Brown had turned around with his hands raised after Wilson shot at his back. According to Dorian Johnson, Wilson then shot Brown multiple times until he fell to the ground, dead.

When I finally got the autopsy report, I learned that Michael Brown had a wound in the back dorsal surface of his forearm that exited from the front of his forearm. He also had a wound in his upper right arm that entered on the volar bicep area and exited from the back of his upper right arm. Both of these wounds had an upward trajectory. He also had a grazing wound across his bicep, and a wound on his right thumb. However, these wounds, in and of themselves, in terms of reconstructing the event, were of little help.

More important, Michael Brown had two gunshot wounds to his chest: one in the midline; the other in his right upper chest, both of which had a downward trajectory. Finally, there were two more shots: one had entered the very top of Michael Brown's head and traveled straight down into his brain and was recovered in the soft tissues of his face; the other, which essentially destroyed his right eye, continued straight down and exited from his jaw. These last two wounds must have occurred with the young man's body in the anatomic position—i.e., perpendicular to the ground. The bullets had traveled in a marked downward trajectory. Now, let's put it all together. I don't mean to be dogmatic, and I recognize differences of opinion, but there's only one way these wounds could have happened.

CNN reported, from video captured at the scene and other information, that all of this took place within 90 seconds, beginning to end, from the time that officer Wilson drove up to Brown and Johnson. Let's say that you are Darren Wilson and I'm Michael Brown. How do I get wounds in my arm going upward? There's only one way. My hands were up. You were standing and I was standing, and you shot me with my arms raised, so the bullet went up and out. You hit me twice, and I began to fall. As I was falling, you shot me twice more in the chest at a downward trajectory. I continued to fall and, as my body became parallel to the ground, "Boom, Boom." The next two shots went straight into the top of my head, and I was found prone, face-down, 30–35 feet from the police car. That's the scenario. If I had been charging you, I would have had to use my hands because I didn't have a weapon.

In the fracas, Officer Wilson was reported to have sustained a blowout fracture of the eye. But when he was released from medical care, there was no indication of such a fracture. Furthermore, video exists showing Wilson, two hours later, in the police station without a mark on his face. It's not close-up, but there's no swelling. He didn't go to the hospital until after that. From where I sit, there was no justification for Officer Wilson's actions, but the police kept talking on TV about "imminent threat." We've heard this before. "We thought his cellphone was a weapon," or some bullshit like that. Michael Brown had no weapon. (With so many video-tapers at the scene, I guess the police didn't have the opportunity to plant anything.)

On TV, a police consultant was saying, "You have to shoot somebody from 21 feet away because, if the person is closer than that, he can be on top of you with a knife or gun in no time." But Michael Brown was 30–35 feet away, so even using their 21-foot rule (of which nobody knows the origin), they fail. Their excuse is nonsense. In Darren Wilson's mind, the only way that he could think of to deal with Michael Brown, who was about 6'5" tall and weighed 290 pounds, was to shoot him. I predicted that there would be a riot, and protesters soon flowed into the streets.

CNN told me that the segment I did about the Michael Brown shooting with Don Lemon, in which I enacted the scenario described above, was the second-most popular segment shown on the network on the day it was broadcast. I gave Lemon the scenario of how I thought the shooting went down, and did it again later with Erin Burnett.

Freddie Gray

The Freddie Gray case, in Baltimore, was fascinating, too, and equally tragic. What was Freddie Gray's crime? He was riding a bicycle, and a cop said he didn't like the way he looked at him. So, the cop went after Freddie, knocked him to the ground, and an altercation ensued as they tried to put him into a police van.

A bystander's video showed Gray, obviously unable to walk, supported by two officers, one on each side, before he was placed in the police van. By that time, I believe that his spinal cord injury had already occurred when the officer chased after him, knocked him down, and leaned on his neck and upper back. So, they put Freddie Gray in the police van, without strapping him down, and did a "joy ride," making four or five other stops before taking him to a hospital. Imagine how Freddie Gray, injured and unrestrained, fared when the cops whipped around corners. When they finally got him to a hospital, he was already quadriplegic, and he died shortly thereafter.

Not long after the incident, I was contacted by the defense attorney for one of the cops involved, an African American officer. I told him that I would like to be of service, but had already spoken out on the case, and I had. I said, "I don't think I can help you." There was no chance that I would work to defend any of the police officers who did what they had done to that young man.

◆ ◆ ◆

When I think back over my career, in addition to the high-profile, I often think of cases that were decidedly less so, yet were equally interesting and, at times, even more exciting. Some took place on the streets of Pittsburgh while others occurred elsewhere. But all allowed me to use my knowledge and experience to right some wrongs and provide some semblance of justice for people of all stripes. What follows are a few of my favorites.

John Charmo

One of my favorite cases involved a man named John Charmo, a Pittsburgh Housing Authority cop. In 1995, he was drawn into a car chase with an African American man named Jerry Jackson (age 44, from Hazelwood) into the Armstrong Tunnel after Jackson had fled from a minor traffic stop. Unbelievably, Charmo wound up shooting Jerry Jackson to death. But was this necessary? He was not a fleeing felon. He didn't hurt or kill anyone. Charmo and his fellow cops said that Jackson was shot after he had turned his car around in the Armstrong Tunnel, and was racing back at them. That story flew for a while, supported by the Allegheny County Coroner who had succeeded me after my first stint in that office.

When I was elected Coroner again in 1996, I said that the explanation offered by the police was sheer nonsense. I was raised only six blocks from the Armstrong tunnel. As a kid, I used to ride my bicycle through it, and remember having difficulty turning my bike around. How could Jerry Jackson have turned a whole car around? I suppose that one could do it after three or four tries, with repeated turns of the wheel. But it's impossible to do so in one swing. The police said, however, that Jackson drove into the tunnel, turned around and came back at them. No way.

The end result was that we had the case reopened. I had the Armstrong Tunnel closed in the middle of the night, and reconstructed the event. We recreated everything and filmed it, and John Charmo, of Glassport, was convicted of involuntary manslaughter. Add this to the collection of cases that did not endear me to some of the local police.

Stephen Scharf

Stephen Scharf and his wife did not have a good relationship. By mutual agreement, both were having affairs. Determined to make a new start, the couple agreed to have a picnic in a place that was familiar to them: just off the Palisades Parkway in New Jersey, overlooking the Hudson River. There, Mrs. Scharf wound up falling off a ledge to her death. Strangely, Mrs. Scharf's body was found 30 or 40 feet beyond the position of the ledge from which she had allegedly fallen. In order for her body to have landed there, authorities surmised, her husband must have thrown her.

The New Jersey State Police, when they reenacted the event, secured themselves carefully as they threw bags of sand from the ledge to see how far away from the ledge they landed. In the trial, prosecution witnesses testified that Stephen, who weighed only about 160 pounds, must have lifted his wife, who weighed at least that much, and tossed her to her death. But when I testified, I said Mr. Scharf would have had to be an 800-pound gorilla to throw his wife's body 30 or 40 feet from the ledge, especially without hurling himself off of the ledge with her.

I visited the ledge from which Stephen Scharf was supposed to have thrown his wife, and it was only about four or five feet wide. Beneath it was another ledge. To move about at all, I had to walk very carefully. Had I thrown anything off that ledge, I would surely have followed it on the long drop downward.

My contention is that Mrs. Scharf had simply fallen from the upper ledge and bounced off the lower one, which sent her body hurling to its final resting place, 30–40 feet away. Nonetheless, the jury believed the cops and proclaimed Stephen Scharf "guilty." I was surprised by that verdict.

The Church of Scientology

In Florida, there had been a minor car accident, so minor that there wasn't a scratch on either party's vehicle; one bumper had just touched the other, moving at about five miles per hour. But a woman in her 30s, who was driving one of the vehicles, got out of her car and proceeded to parade around, completely naked.

The police took the woman to a hospital and it turned out that she was a member

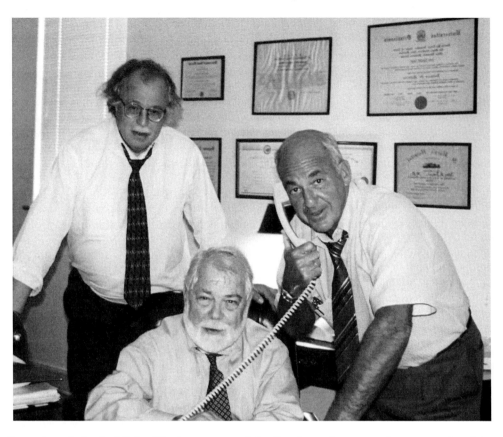

Forensic pathologist Michael Baden, attorney John Feegle, and me consult on a case involving the Church of Scientology, early 1990s.

of the Church of Scientology. Before long, a couple of Church members, who were her friends, came to the woman's aid and wanted to take her "home." They didn't force her to go, nor did they act against medical advice. She simply wanted out, and went with her friends.

They took her to the Church of Scientology's Florida headquarters, which was a former hotel in Clearwater, and it was huge. In a period of years, the Church had all but taken over the city by acquiring real estate and building things of their own. At the headquarters, a Church-employed doctor and nurse did all that they could, but caring for the woman was an overwhelming job. She was urinating and defecating on the floor and wiping it on the walls, and was almost certainly experiencing some kind of psychotic break. That's when I learned that, while Scientologists have no problem with Western medicine, they do not approve of psychiatry, which is what this woman needed desperately. She received 24-hour care but no mental health assistance, and she died.

At first, criminal charges were filed against some individual Church members, and the preliminaries went on for some time. In any event, the Church contacted a man named John Feegle to represent its interests legally. Then I got a call from John. John Feegle and I were good friends. In fact, he had come to testify as a character witness for me in my first corruption trial, in 1980. Interestingly, John had studied to be a priest, but became a forensic pathologist and attorney, like me. (He had been a medical examiner for a while, too.)

Feegle was a sharp guy. As soon as he was contacted by the Church of Scientology, he reached out to consult four or five of the top forensic pathologists in the country. He called me and Michael Baden, and two or three others so that, if we were to be contacted by the prosecution, we would not be available. As it turned out, Michael Baden and I were retained and followed through all the way. We went to the Church's Florida headquarters and met with John Feegle and some representatives of the Church. We had a very structured meeting and, subsequently, worked on the case with John, although he did not remain involved. It ended up being just Baden and me, and we were successful. Criminal charges against the Church members were dropped, but civil lawyers kept pursuing the case, perhaps not realizing that the Church of Scientology had "more money than God" to spend fighting them. What the ultimate outcome of that case was, I do not know.

Miracle Valley

One case of which I'm particularly proud took place in Arizona, in 1982, and involved a black religious community—Christ Miracle Healing Center and Church—and Cochise County. Several incidents with law enforcement, which had been rising in severity, came to a head when local sheriff's deputies, with backup by state law enforcement, attempted to serve bench warrants for the arrest of three members of the Church.

On October 23, authorities rolled into the Church's compound in Miracle Valley, a traditionally white community until the Church moved in, with a single sheriff's car, attempting but ultimately failing to locate the persons for whom the bench warrants were issued. Soon, another car drove up filled with angry Church members. Feeling threatened, the deputies on-site called for backup support, which was tantamount to a small army, including 17 cars and 35 deputies. Soon, an estimated 150 Church members—men, women and children—began attacking the deputies with sticks, rocks, pipes, lumber, garden rakes, knives and firearms, and shots were fired from multiple weapons, on both sides.

After being attacked, Sheriff Deputy Ray Thatcher, who was the designated SWAT sniper for the authorities on that day, fired a semi-automatic rifle killing two Church members, whom he said were preparing to fire directly at him. During the shootout, which lasted about 15 minutes, an estimated 20 Church members, allegedly armed with sticks and guns, surrounded the deputies and forced them to retreat. In the melee, beside the two Church members who were killed by Deputy Thatcher, seven police officers were injured. One wounded Church member and one wounded police officer later died.

Criminal charges were brought against 19 Church members for their alleged part in the shootout. I went out there, conducted an investigation, and determined that the fatal shots all struck the victims from the side or the rear, and that it was not possible to conclude from which direction the other, non-fatal shots were fired, or in what order they were fired. I also determined that the forensic-science evidence scientifically repudiated Deputy Thatcher's accounts of the shooting. I met with the local prosecutor at the request of the defense attorney and reviewed in great detail my reconstruction of the event. Shortly thereafter, all homicide charges against the Church members were withdrawn.

Mario Madrigal, Jr.

Another case of which I'm very proud took place in Arizona also—in Mesa, to be exact. In August 2003, a 14-year-old boy named Mario Madrigal, Jr., reportedly had been carrying on and was out of control. So, his mother, Martha Madrigal, an Hispanic woman, called the police for help. In short order, the boy was shot by the police multiple times, and was killed.

I did a second autopsy on the Madrigal boy and consulted in this matter with my colleague, Dr. Henry Lee. In August 2004, Martha and Mario Madrigal, Sr., then husband and wife, filed a "wrongful death" action against the City of Mesa and, eventually, won a big settlement. Our review and analysis succeeded in reversing the likely end result of the Madrigal family's tragedy, i.e., no indictments would come down for the police officers involved. This was a tragic death of a child that was completely unjustified. Henry and I proved that the prosecution's expert, a criminalist named Lucien Haag, had "reconstructed" a total fabrication of the event.

Anthony Proviano

In December 1997, Anthony Proviano, a 29-year-old medical student, was headed home to celebrate Christmas with his family in Baldwin Borough, Pennsylvania, when he stopped at a hotel in Belmont County, Ohio. On December 28, his body was found in heavy brush about a quarter-mile from the hotel, on an abandoned township road. He died from a single gunshot to the chest, and the authorities signed the death out as a suicide with no autopsy. The Proviano family was stunned. They refused to accept the decision and called on me to look into the matter for them.

The private autopsy showed no traces of gunpowder residue on Anthony's hands, but a determination was made that he had shot himself. After a year of the Provianos pushing police and politicians from two states to act, the Ohio coroner finally relented, reluctantly, and listed the cause of Anthony Proviano's death as "undetermined." In 2001, after reviewing my consultation report, in which I explained why this shooting was a murder and not an accident or a suicide, a new coroner in Belmont County changed the determination of Anthony's death to "homicide."

In the end, with the aid of more in-depth investigation and information from the news media, the perpetrator of the crime, a woman, was arrested. She was subsequently tried and convicted in 2006 for the murder of Anthony Proviano, and died in prison three years later at the age of 53.

Lisa Lambert

On December 20, 1991, Laurie Show, a 16-year-old sophomore student at Conestoga Valley High School, lay dying in her home in Lancaster, Pennsylvania, with her vocal cords cut. Show's mother, Hazel, who had discovered her severely injured daughter after returning home from a meeting at Laurie's school, reported to the police that her daughter had named Lisa Lambert as her killer.

Lisa had been harassing Laurie Show after learning that Laurie had briefly dated a young man named Lawrence "Butch" Yunkin over the summer. Butch had dated Lisa before his relationship with Laurie, and the two had resumed their relationship immediately after Butch and Laurie's breakup because Lisa was carrying Butch's child. Laurie Show reported to her mother that, while she was seeing Yunkin, he had date-raped her, which upped the ante for Lisa Lambert, Laurie's harasser.

Lisa was present when the murder happened, so the DA, as they often do, chose to go after her, and she was arrested, tried and convicted in 1992 for Laurie Show's murder. Lisa Lambert received "life in prison without parole," as did her friend Tabitha Buck, her convicted accomplice. Butch Yunkin received a lesser sentence for his testimony and was granted parole in 2003.

I became involved when members of the news media asked me to speak about the case. It featured some fascinating medical testimony about whether or not someone with slashed vocal cords could audibly vocalize. Nonetheless, Lisa remained in prison, even after an appeal led to a retrial in 1997, which resulted in a finding of "prosecutorial misconduct" during her initial trial. Unfortunately for Lisa, that ruling was overturned in January 1998 by a federal appeals panel.

In jail, Lisa has earned a college degree, with high honors, and wrote a book about her case. I had been corresponding with her on and off, trying to help her at different times, but to no avail. Do I think she's ever going to be released? Probably not.

◆ ◆ ◆

I could go on and on about interesting cases in which I've been involved, locally and nationally, over the years. However, I would like to take a moment to apprise you of a host of international cases that have called on my experience and expertise in search of resolutions.

The Bahamas

One day, in the Bahamas, a young woman was reported missing. In the process of searching for her, authorities found a body. But it turned out not to be that of the young woman in question, but rather another who had not been reported missing but who, upon inquiry, was missing indeed. After the first body was found, Bahamian law enforcement kept searching and found a second, and called me for help.

The missing girl they called me about was from the U.S.; the other was from Britain. Both bodies were found essentially skeletonized in a beach area, and the authorities asked me to do the autopsies. So, I examined both bodies and identified them anthropologically. (One woman had a hip implant with a metal screw on which the manufacturer's name was stamped.) Then I studied the police reports and determined the cause of death in both cases was "homicide."

The authorities searched the islands and located a native Bahamian; a young, black man who sold trinkets on the beach. He appeared harmless and, apparently, was intellectually challenged, but not severely so. He was not the criminal type, but the police had information about him that was enough to make an arrest.

I traveled to the Bahamas and testified at the preliminary hearing and trial for one victim, and then at the preliminary hearing and trial for the other, too. By the third time I went down there, when I walked into the courtroom, the defendant said, "Hi, Dr. Wecht"—and soon was convicted.

The Bahamians were pleased and grateful. Henry Lee says that I am now a legend in the islands.

On January 16, 2020, I arrived at my office to find an email from the Honorable Justice Bernard Turner of the Bahamian Supreme Court *"Dr. Wecht, I still remember the names of the young victims of those awful murders, and we remain grateful for your assistance all those years ago... If you ever need a mid-winter break from those cooler temperatures, the Bahamas would be happy to see you, under better circumstances. Yours sincerely, Bernard."* It's nice to be remembered and appreciated.

Daniel and Anna Nicole Smith

While we're in the Bahamas, let's talk about Daniel Smith, model and Playboy Playmate Anna Nicole Smith's teenage son. The request for my involvement came from Howard Stern; not the radio shock-jock, but rather Anna Nicole's attorney, who was also her significant other or, at least, her living companion. (He claimed that the two had been married.)

I was somewhere out West when I received the call from Mr. Stern. I was needed in the Bahamas right away, but I didn't have my passport. It was not long after all the nonsense had started with my federal trial in Pittsburgh, so I had to get special permission to leave the U.S. I also had to get a short-term work permit from the Department of Immigration in the Bahamas.

In the Bahamas, I did the autopsy on Daniel Smith, and concurred with local authorities that his death, on September 10, 2006, was due to a drug overdose. On "Larry King Live," I stated that Daniel had died from a lethal combination of the antidepressants Zoloft and Lexapro, and methadone, the latter of which is used to treat heroin addiction and chronic pain.

I was subsequently consulted on the death of Anna Nicole herself, who died unexpectedly on February 8, 2007, at a hotel in Hollywood, Florida, also from a prescription drug overdose. I wound up not doing the autopsy because her body had become decomposed by then. In my opinion, there was no foul play connected to her death, and I don't think there was negligence. There was no question about Anna Nicole's cause of

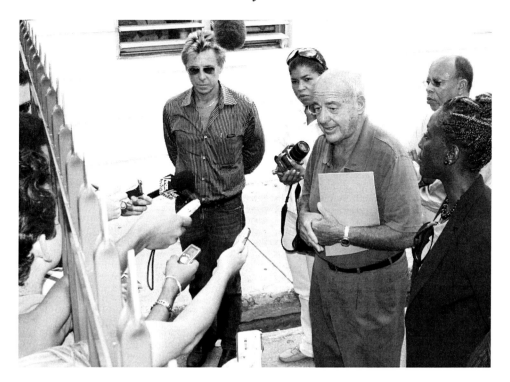

Nassau, Bahamas, September 2006. Talking to the media about the autopsy of Daniel Wayne Smith, the 26-year-old son of actress Anna Nicole Smith (*Associated Press*).

death being due to drugs, just like her son. The only question about Daniel Smith is, from where did the drugs come? It was looked into, but no one could establish that the drugs came from Howard Stern, or anyone else in particular.

Israel

I have been consulted on two cases in Israel, one of which was a prosecution for murder involving an on-duty guard at a kibbutz who was accused of causing the death of a teenage boy. Reportedly, some Arab teenagers were yelling and throwing stones, and were warned to stop and go away. They didn't stop, and kept approaching, so a guard chased them away. During the chase, one of the Arab boys was injured, and was taken to a hospital but sadly, he died.

An autopsy was done and the medical examiner, an Israeli, said that the boy had been struck by the guard and called it "murder." The case boiled down to a question of whether or not the guard had struck the boy or whether the boy had simply fallen.

At the request of the guard's family, I went to Israel and to the scene of the boy's death and studied everything, in addition to reviewing the autopsy report. I concluded that the nature of the injury definitely indicated that it was from a fall and not from a blow. The judge, a woman, spoke English, and I was permitted to do so also, as I don't speak Hebrew. I testified at great length, explaining all that I could, and the guard was acquitted of homicide charges. In the Israeli justice system, they don't hesitate to investigate sensitive cases, and don't try to cover them up. The police had been mistaken, and the matter was then resolved.

For my second, and much weirder, case in Israel, I received a call from an attorney representing the family of a young Romanian-Jewish immigrant who was conscripted into the Israel Defense Forces (IDF), and didn't like it. His regiment was on a march one day, and he kept complaining. The march continued and, when the sergeant looked back, the young man wasn't there. He sent two soldiers to look for him and they found the young man, dead.

The IDF determined that the young man had shot himself, and wanted an autopsy to be performed. The family protested, so no autopsy was done, and the body was buried. Then the family members themselves dug up the young man's remains and took them to their home. They were relatively poor people and lived in a government building, with no air-conditioning, yet they kept a dead body on the premises. The family told the authorities that, if they made a move to come and take the body, they would be hurt or killed by way of a set of explosive charges that had been set up around the home.

Negotiations ensued, and the family agreed to have the body relocated to an air-conditioned facility. They lived near Be'er Sheva, in the Negev desert part of southern Israel, not far from David Ben-Gurion's own kibbutz, Sde Boker. The hospital there included an old portion that was no longer in use, but had a refrigerated cooler. The body would be kept there, in a small building, which had a little courtyard and stood apart from the other buildings. There, the family began preparing for a 24-hour per day vigil. Nevertheless, I was called to come over and do an autopsy.

My plane landed, and after it had pulled to a stop, an IDF officer came aboard. He was a major, and it turned out that he was also an attorney. He wanted to fill me in on the background of the case. So, we talked and then deplaned. When I arrived at the terminal, I was looking for someone to guide me to where I was needed. I didn't see anyone, but heard some yelling and screaming. "What's going on?" I thought. It turned out that the mother of the dead soldier was there and had the news media following her, along with the lawyer who called me originally. She was claiming that the Israeli government, specifically the army, had boarded the airplane to influence me in some way. I did not know that the major was going to board the plane and ask to speak with me. The military lawyer said that the woman's claims were ridiculous, and that I should ignore them.

We traveled to where the young man's body was located, a three- or four-hour drive, and I woke up early the next morning to do the autopsy. The family was present, and the body had been taken out. But then, suddenly, the family decided that they didn't want me to do an autopsy after all. Apparently, they didn't trust me. So, I went back to the hotel and called my Israeli contact. He asked me to write everything up, and I did. I sat down and wrote a seven- or eight-page report, longhand. Subsequently, I learned that Dr. Michael Baden had been called, but backed off as well when they found out that he was Jewish. Jews are "contaminated," don't you know? Is that what their problem was with me, too? I found out later that the dead man's family finally accepted a Scandinavian pathologist, one of those international liberals, who confirmed that it was a suicide.

Kuwait

One day, I got a call from a New York attorney who worked for one of the largest investigative groups in the world. They were preparing to conduct investigations following the invasion of Kuwait by Iraq, the action that led to the Persian Gulf War and Operation Desert Storm in 1990.

After we whipped the asses of the Iraqi military and drove them out of Kuwait, allied forces, including those from the U.S., learned that Iraqi soldiers had gone into a hospital in Kuwait and removed newborn infants from incubators—not to kill the babies, per se, but to steal the state-of-the-art equipment. What happened to the babies? They were all killed and buried. A British outfit in Kuwait, using ground sonar, located the remains of the infants beneath the ground.

We reviewed all the evidence and were set to go when the effort was canceled at the last minute by the U.S. government. I believe they knew that, if it came out that the Iraqis had killed babies, the American public would not have accepted George H.W. Bush's decision to pull out and allow Saddam Hussein to stay in power. The operation was, politically, way too hot to handle. This was not the first time (nor will it be the last) that government officials have intruded into a medical-legal investigation for political reasons, usually to avoid an autopsy being performed or to have an autopsy conducted by a pathologist who could be manipulated.

Australia

Henry Lee was contacted on referral from the United Nations about a woman who was looking into the death of her husband. Australians were alarmed that numerous aborigines had died by suicidal hanging while in jail on relatively minor charges. Many believed that they had been murdered.

Henry contacted me and Michael Baden and we met in Connecticut to talk with a widow of one of the victims. She was a strong, dynamic and articulate woman who was pursuing the situation aggressively. We reviewed the cases and felt that some serious questions had been raised. We were ready to go to Australia to do exhumation autopsies, but those plans fell through. Our reports, however, were filed and I wound up testifying, formally, before a judge via a long-distance setup. The Australian government then launched a formal investigation into these cases.

Argentina

Alberto Nisman was an Argentinian lawyer who worked as a federal prosecutor and was the chief investigator of the 1994 car bombing of the Jewish Center in Buenos Aires, which killed 85 people. It was the worst terrorist attack in Argentina's history.

On January 18, 2015, Nisman was found dead at his home, one day before he was scheduled to report his findings, with supposedly incriminating evidence against high-ranking officials of the Argentinian government, including former President Cristina Fernández de Kirchner. An Argentinian television station called and asked if I would review the case. A news team came to Pittsburgh from Buenos Aires and interviewed me at great length. I said that, to me, the case looked like a murder.

The resulting film became the number one TV program in Buenos Aires at the time. The official ruling was that Nisman had committed suicide and, despite implorations and challenges, the government stood by it. Two years later, the case was finally ruled a murder. The official scenario that was played out in court portrayed the details of Nisman's death just as I had explained in my TV interview.

Brazil

One day, I was contacted by a man who worked for a large international company with a branch in Brazil. The company was planning to build a hydroelectric dam in Peru, and two engineers were dispatched to pick the best site for the project. So, the engineers traveled to a Peruvian outpost to choose a location, but there was no happiness among the locals, who feared that their habitat would be destroyed by a large, modern project.

The engineers were middle-aged, healthy, intelligent guys, and they knew what they were doing. But soon, one engineer said, "I'm tired. It's too hot. I'm going to wait here," at a little trading post; a "last-chance-to-buy-a-drink-and-take-a-piss" type of place. So, the other team members went off to do their jobs, but when they returned, the engineer who stayed behind was nowhere to be found. At that point, the other engineer who was in charge said, "I'll go and find him." He went out—and never returned. The others searched, but didn't find either man.

The next day, after some discussion, the team searched again, and found the bodies of both engineers, with no apparent injuries. Autopsies were conducted but didn't reveal anything. The bodies were then sent back to Brazil where second autopsies were performed and, still, nothing.

Later on, a young man came to Pittsburgh and brought me a load of materials related to the case, and I looked through it. He had spent a lot of time on this, and subsequently provided some additional materials, which I sent off for toxicological analysis. The bottom line was that I never could find the cause of death. The bodies had no injuries and no disease processes. It came down to two possibilities: It was very hot, the engineers got lost, and became dehydrated; or, it was possible that they had been poisoned by a substance that none of our usual toxicological tests could detect, the kind of poison used by indigenous tribes like the ones living in that territory.

I believe that it was an organic substance, but I could never prove it. You can't test for most kinds of biological poisons because they readily metabolize and decompose in the body, and they also don't necessarily show, even after testing with highly sophisticated toxicological equipment. The engineers could have ingested something that was put into their food or water, but who knows? The case was bizarre and I don't know its outcome, but I do know that no criminal charges were ever filed against anybody. It was a fascinating case and a very frustrating one, too, because I couldn't come up with anything. There I was, consulted and paid, but could provide no resolution. I was disappointed intellectually and professionally by this matter, and I'm not really used to that.

Singapore and the Philippines

Lee Kuan Yew was the Prime Minister of Singapore and governed there for decades. He is recognized as the nation's "founding father," and led the country's transition from Third World to First World status in a single generation, after the nation broke away from Britain following World War II.

In 2002, I was invited to Singapore as the 55th distinguished scholar hosted since the time the honors program had been established. (Thirty-eight of the recipients had been Nobel Prize winners.) I gave 18 lectures about forensic pathology in two weeks, and spoke to medical, legal, law enforcement and academic groups. My wife, Sigrid, and I were wined and dined, and put up in a beautiful penthouse suite. We each had our own car and driver, and were fed unbelievable 18-course meals. It was the "big time," but it would not be my last visit to that incredible country.

Years later, in Singapore, a Filipino maid who was working for a wealthy Chinese family was found dead, along with a three- or four-year-old boy from the family with whom she lived and worked. Another Filipino maid who worked for another wealthy Chinese family there was ultimately charged with the murders after the authorities learned that the dead maid had refused to lend money to the other, and they got into a fight. The killer was tried, found "guilty" and executed. In Singapore, when it comes to meting out justice, they don't mess around. I was not involved in that case at all, but stay with me.

Before the killer-maid was executed, the Filipino government implored Singapore's leadership not to do it. The case had become a controversial political issue in the Philippines, which was in the middle of a national election, and somebody was playing this case for all it was worth. The country was ready to break diplomatic relations with Singapore over it. Here's where I came in.

I was contacted by the medical examiner of Singapore, with whom I had become friends. His name was Professor Chao Tzee Cheng, and he called on me, Michael Baden and Henry Lee. The dispute had reached such a crescendo that the body of the dead maid was exhumed, and a Filipino pathologist had concluded that the injuries she sustained were such that they could only have been inflicted by a strong male or by someone trained in the martial arts. We stated that there was no way that the woman who had been tried, convicted, and executed could have committed that murder.

We flew to Singapore and had a special meeting with Chao to review the case. We then flew to Manila the next day, were picked up at the airport, and learned that this case had become a big deal in the Philippines. We went to the penthouse floor of a hospital and present were about 20 Filipino doctors of different kinds. They were very friendly and hospitable, and were impressed by Michael Baden, Henry Lee and me (a "dream team" of sorts). They presented the skeletal remains of the deceased maid to us because the body had decomposed. We examined everything and concluded that some of the things that the Filipino pathologist had diagnosed were clearly postmortem artifacts from decomposition. Then we left there at one or two in the morning.

Before we left, however, we participated in a huge news conference, which was attended by at least 50 television, radio and newspaper reporters, and calmly stated our findings, after which we returned to the Embassy of Singapore in Manila. It was late, and we were hungry, so we had a bite to eat. Then Chao, my friend, said, "Get some sleep and we'll see you in the morning. We're going to fly back to Singapore tomorrow, and then you can go home."

Five or six hours later, we awoke, prepared to leave and, guess what? The place was empty. The issue was so hot that our hosts feared that they were in jeopardy of serious physical harm. They knew that nothing would be done to us Americans, of course. So, a government plane had flown them all out in the middle of the night. Chao and all the rest were gone.

Pakistan

One day, I got a call from a man who worked for the World Bank. He came to Pittsburgh and wanted to meet and talk with me. His brother, who had been chief of staff for the Pakistan Armed Forces, had died suddenly at home and was buried according to Islamic Law, with no autopsy, after which allegations were made that he had been poisoned. Somehow, the man felt comfortable with me, and the case became a major political issue. If his brother had been poisoned during election season, the political ramifications would have been horrendous. But who would have poisoned him?

The authorities decided to exhume the body, and the family was in agreement. They brought in three pathologists: me, somebody recommended by Scotland Yard, and someone from Sûreté, the top-level police agency in France. We didn't know each other, but we met and spoke with a high-ranking official in Islamabad and, the next morning, flew in a private military helicopter about 60 miles or so south. The dead man's family was wealthy and had their own burial ground where he had been laid to rest. We were to conduct the exhumation there.

It was 110 degrees under the canopy, which was something to experience. We dug up the body, which had been buried in a good coffin and very deep. Amazingly, it was well preserved. So, we did an autopsy. We all took tissue samples separately and the process went smoothly. Then we returned home and submitted our reports independently. Toxicology findings were negative and we all concurred that there was evidence of significant coronary artery disease. Our findings were accepted, and that ended the controversy.

China

A student studying in China was found dead, secluded in a bathroom. He had apparently sealed off all possible areas of entry and egress, and asphyxiated himself. It was deemed a suicide, but an autopsy was done. The Chinese translated the report for me, I reviewed its findings, and concurred. Nothing suggested foul play.

When a person is trapped in a closed, sealed space for enough time, he will lose consciousness. I believe that the student had neither the means nor the courage to inflict bodily harm on himself, so he barricaded himself in a bathroom, sealed it tight and suffocated himself. It would have been difficult for him to gather enough pills in China to do the job. But he could have thrown himself in front of a truck, jumped out of a building or hanged himself. That's how we do it in the West.

Taiwan

In my career, I have worked on three cases in Taiwan. The first involved a young man who had just been granted a junior faculty position at Carnegie Mellon University (CMU), in Pittsburgh. Apparently, he was a native of Taiwan, and he, his wife and newborn baby went to visit their families before starting the academic year. Unfortunately, the local security police picked up the young man one night for questioning. The next thing his family knew, he had "jumped off" a building on the campus of National Taiwan University. The young man's death was signed out as a suicide.

Soon thereafter, I received a call from Richard Cyert, then President of CMU, who asked if I would go to Taiwan and do an autopsy on his former junior faculty member. Of course, I said yes. A CMU professor, a very nice guy by the name of Morris H. DeGroot, went with me. Fortunately, the Taiwanese had kept the young man's body frozen, and I did an autopsy. I went to the scene where the body had been found. I laid it all out and concluded that the death could not have been a suicide. The young man's body had to have been thrown. So, we had a meeting with some Taiwanese officials to whom I explained everything. They eventually concluded that the death was a murder and changed the death certificate.

For Taiwanese case number two, Sigrid went with me. This case was political. It seemed that the "grand old man" of the aboriginal Nationalist Party, which had been suppressed and outlawed by Chiang Kai-shek, turned up dead, with injuries. The man lived alone, in hermit-like fashion, and was revered by the people of the small, island nation. Interestingly, the native Taiwanese people are Chinese by default. They are not actually Chinese. They see themselves as Formosans, an indigenous people who have lived on the island of Taiwan long before it became occupied by China's Qing Dynasty in 1683 and, later, by the Japanese Empire in 1895.

Anyway, the family called and wanted me to do an autopsy to determine the cause of the old man's death. I remember that his daughter was an executive at the second-largest city down from Taipei, and we went there to pay our respects. Then we went back to the location where the man had died: a two-story building where he had a huge room, with newspapers piled up to the ceiling.

Knowing that we were present, the news media turned out in droves. Taiwanese journalists make the American media look like child's play. It was unbelievable. They came with their theories, based on nothing, saying that maybe somebody came in from the roof, through the window, and killed him. So, I went up to the roof and walked around, checking things out. It was known that, on the day he died, the old man had been to a party, and I believe that he got drunk and came home, stumbled and hit his head on the edge of his bureau. I was completely honest as I shared my thoughts. In the meantime, the media was clamoring for an autopsy. In retrospect, I realize that I should not have spoken to anyone about my preliminary findings.

Soon, the autopsy was set. Everybody was in place. The body was on the autopsy table, and I had the scalpel in my hand when I heard someone yelling. The old man's son, who was a member of the national legislature, decided that he didn't want an autopsy to be conducted after all. So, it didn't happen. I still believe that the old man's death was an accident, but others believe that he had been murdered because he did have a serious head injury. I can understand that. But, for political reasons, the family decided, after learning of my preliminary investigative findings, that it was better not to have an autopsy performed and simply leave the allegations of murder alone.

Now, for Taiwanese case number three, and more political intrigue… I was in California with Dr. Henry Lee on the Scott Peterson case, doing the second autopsy of Scott's deceased wife Laci, when Henry received a call. He was needed in Taiwan immediately. There had been an attempt to assassinate the president of Taiwan on the day before the national election. Down in the polls, the president was campaigning in an open car. His vice president, a woman, was seated to his left when shots were fired. She was hit in the knee and the president was struck in the abdomen, but they both survived.

Henry had an engagement of great importance and couldn't go to Taiwan immediately, so he asked me if I would go and I said, "Certainly." I cleared my schedule and went with two other people: Henry's right-hand man, who was a former Connecticut state trooper, and an expert criminalist from Arizona. We went to the scene of the shooting and reenacted everything. We examined the car, which had been sequestered in a garage. We went to the hospital and spoke with the doctors and nurses who had treated the president and vice president after the incident. We covered everything in two or three days. Then we went to the president's palace, where he graciously received us.

There we were, sitting in the presidential palace, talking about a bunch of things; and then we got into the shooting. The controversy had become increasingly intense, and the president wound up winning re-election by the smallest of margins. His opponents were screaming that he had staged the assassination attempt to get public attention and the "sympathy vote." They contended that he had never been shot or wounded. But shots were fired, and the vice president had, indeed, caught a bullet in the knee, and they couldn't explain that away.

So, we were sitting there, graciously and comfortably, for 20 minutes at least when, all of a sudden, the president stands, pulls up his shirt, unbuckles his belt and pulls down his pants for us to look at his wound. Indeed, there was one, which had healed a bit, but it showed the linear streaking across the abdomen that correlated with what had been reported to us by the doctors at the hospital. There was no question that the president had been shot. And his wound, had it been a half-inch deeper, could have been fatal. Yet the controversy continued. The President's opponents even alleged that he had shot himself. But the weapon involved was found. It was a homemade contraption.

◆ ◆ ◆

MARK GERAGOS: *There was a case where I was dealing with a young man who was charged with murder. Cyril pointed me in the right direction and the jury, ultimately, ended up hung. Without his direction, that client would have been convicted and sentenced to life. Cyril got me thinking about the case in a way that I hadn't before, and I give him credit for effectively allowing me to hang that jury 6–6.*

So, do I ever get the feeling that I might have made a mistake on a case? Absolutely. Medicine is not an absolute science, and that includes the most tangible, concrete scientific branch of medicine, which is pathology. Pathology, by definition, is more concrete because you can hold the tissue, look at it under a microscope, and do tests on it. But even pathology is not an absolute science. There have been times when my opinion was wrong. I'm not embarrassed by that. I can only say that I try to call things as I see them, but I am not infallible when I give an opinion. I remember that, at some point, I'm going to be deposed. An attorney is going to ask me a lot of probing questions and, after everything, I must enter the courtroom to testify, so I have to know my stuff.

JOHN PECK: *Cyril is extremely impartial and independent. He goes where the facts lead him and bases his conclusions and his findings on what the facts are. I doubt that anybody has ever [successfully] challenged his integrity in terms of pathology or as an expert witness.*

I remember working with John Peck, the DA of Westmoreland County, Pennsylvania, on a case in which a podiatrist was accused of killing his wife by suffocating her. The defense said that the defendant had fainted during a struggle with his wife, who fainted at the same time, and that he caused her death accidentally by falling on top of her on the bed where the struggle took place.

JOHN PECK: *Cyril's analysis was that this couldn't have happened because there are certain effects that are different from what they call "compression suffocation," when you have somebody on top of you, as opposed to ordinary suffocation, whereby you can't breathe through your mouth or nose. The jury believed Cyril, that this had been an intentional killing. That was a significant case, too. I think the defense had hired Henry Lee, as well as another pathologist, to examine the evidence, and they mounted a significant effort. But Cyril's the person we go to. We don't try to find anybody other than him. There's nobody else that we care to use. Who else has such a local, national and international reputation? There is no one better.*

Respected public servants such as John Peck appreciate my thoroughness and willingness to explain my findings on a level that everybody can understand.

JOHN PECK: *Cyril doesn't talk down to jurors. He's a good teacher. He takes his time. He supports all of his opinions with facts and in a language that's very understandable. He can explain something extremely complicated of a medical nature in layman's terms and in a way that the jury trusts. I don't find him in any way flashy or wanting the spotlight. He appears humble on the witness stand. When his opinions are challenged, he remains independent, impartial, unbiased, and never hostile to the person who is challenging him. He is accommodating and accessible to those of us who need him. I don't know what we would do without him.*

Two Final Cases—And a Point

Rebecca Zahau

Rebecca Zahau had been discovered dead on July 13, 2011, at the Spreckels Mansion in Coronado, California, where she lived with her multi-millionaire boyfriend, Jonah Shacknai, CEO of Medicis Pharmaceutical. Earlier, on July 11, Shacknai's six-year-old son, Max, had fallen from a staircase banister and suffered multiple, life-threatening injuries while in the care of Rebecca and her 13-year-old sister, in the same beachfront mansion. On July 16, little Max Shacknai died due to brain damage caused by oxygen deprivation resulting from his injuries. His death was ruled accidental.

The day after Max's accident, Rebecca made a trip to the local airport to bid farewell to her sister, who flew back to Missouri, and picked up her boyfriend's brother, Adam Shacknai, who had just arrived in San Diego from Memphis, Tennessee. After dinner with Adam and Rebecca, Jonah Shacknai went to keep vigil at Max's bedside with Max's mother, from whom he was divorced. Adam Shacknai returned with Rebecca to the beach house, where he would spend the night.

On the morning of July 13, around 6:48, Adam placed a 9-1-1 call to the San Diego police stating that he had found Rebecca nude, hanging from a balcony, with her wrists and ankles bound tightly behind her back. (He had cut her body down before the police arrived.) In short order, the sheriff signed out the death as a suicide, and members of the Zahau family were outraged. A neighbor had reported hearing someone screaming around the time of Rebecca Zahau's death.

Soon, I was consulted by the Zahau family, conducted an exhumation autopsy on Rebecca's body for them, and offered lengthy depositions several times. I also appeared on the "Dr. Phil" TV program to discuss the case and my findings. Indeed, Rebecca's hands were clasped behind her back and her calves were tied so tightly that she actually had bruising on her inner calf muscles. She had a ligature around her neck, which ran across the master bedroom floor and was attached to a bedpost, and a shirt-sleeve was stuffed into her mouth. The balcony's balustrade was about 4'6" feet high, and Rebecca was only 5'2". Given this fact, and all the binding, how could she have thrown herself over the balustrade?

The defense tried to say, with no proof at all, that Rebecca Zahau had committed suicide because she felt guilty that the little boy suffered his fall while she was look-ing after him. But, as a matter of fact, she had been interviewed by a police psycholo-gist after the incident, because the police were concerned about her state of mind. She checked out fine. Nevertheless, the medical examiner, sheriff, and district attorney in San Diego continued to insist that Rebecca Zahau's death was a suicide, and refused to budge on that point, notwithstanding the Zahau family's many appeals. Soon, the family hired an attorney, Keith Greer, and, in a matter of days before the statute of limitations ran out on a civil action, the Zahaus filed a "wrongful death" suit, accusing Jonah Shacknai's brother, Adam, a tugboat operator (who would have been very handy at tying and binding things), of being responsible for Rebecca's death.

Adam Shacknai's chief legal counsel, who was being paid for by his multi-millionaire brother, was Dan K. Webb, a well-known lawyer (and former U.S. Attorney) from Chi-cago who had been involved in several major national cases. I testified for the Zahau family, and was thoroughly cross-examined by Dan Webb, for roughly three hours. I stated that the hyoid bone fracture in Rebecca's throat was caused by manual strangula-tion, not by suicidal hanging. Therefore, I considered Rebecca's death a homicide. The jury must have agreed with my testimony—that Adam Shacknai murdered Rebecca Zahau—contrary to the San Diego medical examiner's official ruling of "suicide." As a result, they came back with a verdict of $5.2 million for the Zahaus.

I believe that the San Diego police turned their backs because of the grieving fa-ther's status. They didn't give a damn about Rebecca Zahau, or her family. I was very proud of this case and am happy that it was resolved, at least, in civil court. Postscript: Keith Greer, the Zahau family's attorney during Adam Shacknai's trial, told the jury, "We're not in this for the money." In fact, the Zahaus had previously turned down an offer of $1.5 million to settle the matter. They just wanted to get the truth out that Re-becca would not have committed suicide.

Lonnie Swartz

In October 2012, Lonnie Swartz, a U.S. Border Patrol agent, responded, in what he called self-defense, by firing 16 gunshots through the border fence that separates Arizona from Mexico, because rocks—baseball-sized, and bigger—were being thrown at him from the Mexican side.

José Antonio Elena Rodríguez, 16, died four blocks from his home in Nogales, Mexico, after being hit 10 times by Swartz's gunfire. The U.S. government contended that Rodríguez was not throwing rocks at the time he was gunned down. In fact, they said, he was running away before being knocked to the ground by the agent's barrage of bullets, and shot in the head by Swartz while the boy was still alive. As a result, federal prosecutors charged Border Patrol agent Swartz with homicide. The major issue had to do with the position of the boy. Was he still running, or was he shot when he was lying down? The government believed that they could prove the latter, with a little help.

I was consulted on the case, and reviewed everything. But in addition to the opin-ion of the local medical examiner, the prosecution reached out to Emma Lew, the Chief

Medical Examiner of Dade County/Miami, Florida. Dr. Lew is a very competent foren-sic pathologist, and in her deposition, she offered a strong opinion. My deposition went on for five or six hours. After all, this was a very, very complex, protracted, and highly controversial case. Then I went to testify.

It was April of 2018. I gave my testimony and the defense attorneys were delighted. I explained that the issue was really Dr. Lew, who claimed that she could reconstruct the exact position of the shooter, the exact position of the victim, the sequence of the shots, and, hence, the trajectory, angle and range of fire of every single shot. That was bullshit, as it was in the Menendez brothers' case. The jury understood it was bullshit in Menendez, and they understood it was bullshit here, too. Lonnie Swartz was found "not guilty" of second-degree murder, but jurors were deadlocked on whether or not he was guilty of manslaughter. Prosecutors vowed to try Swartz again, this time on lesser charges of voluntary and involuntary manslaughter.

I was consulted again by the defense attorneys representing Lonnie Swartz in the October 2018 retrial. Trying the case for the government was Assistant U.S. Attorney Wallace Kleindienst (incidentally, the son of Richard Nixon's Attorney General, Rich-ard G. Kleindienst). I was deposed for a second time, for another five or six hours, and went back and testified on the manslaughter issue. In his opening argument, Klein-dienst said that Swartz came ready to shoot. He had drawn his gun before he even got to the scene. However, no one else who responded to the rock-throwing had drawn their weapons.

I testified for the better part of a day and was asked, among other questions, "When a rock the size of a baseball is hurled, what would be the degree of force if it struck someone? Could a rock of that size kill a person if it hit them?" "You're damn right it could," I said. The jury wasn't out very long. This second time around, the jurors found Lonnie Swartz "not guilty" of involuntary manslaughter, but did not reach a verdict on the more serious charge of voluntary manslaughter. The Feds then elected not to pro-ceed further with the case.

I realize and often say that the cases on which I consult are not about me. I'm just a witness. I'm just one component. On the Swartz case, it wasn't for me to get into the training or the psychology of the U.S. Border Patrol. I dealt with the pathology of the incident. Those rocks constituted potentially lethal weapons, and Emma Lew couldn't prove what she alleged.

Although it was a civil matter, on the other side of the Zahau case was the chief medical examiner of San Diego, who was a very prominent professional. (Subsequently, he became chief medical examiner of Los Angeles.) In the Swartz case, I testified oppo-site local forensic pathologists, and they even brought in the chief medical examiner of Dade County/Miami, Florida. She was their witness in that trial, yet I prevailed. Don't forget that, when I go to work on out-of-state cases, I'm a "foreigner." The reason I refer to this is because I want to make a point, even though it might sound egotistical. It's a fact that, within a period of several months, I testified in two cases with top forensic pathologists and medical examiners on the other side, and in both instances, I came out on top. There is nothing magical. I don't hypnotize juries. I just thoroughly review each case and look at the facts. I do research, discuss it with the attorneys, and prepare. And then I testify. I come across as credible, articulate without embellishment, and firm, but not overly dramatic. I explain things in terms that juries can comprehend, even highly technical issues.

◆ ◆ ◆

I'm proud of the fact that I started doing consultations at the beginning of my career, and that I'm still getting consultations from all over the world today, 60 years later. If I had been a shyster, a charlatan, or somebody who just plowed forward, loudly proclaiming this and that without the support of science, how long do you think it would have taken before I was uncovered and shot down? I'm a medical-legal consultant and before you get to my expertise, experience and credentials, you run into my credibility. I've been doing this for a long time, with great success.

MICHAEL WELNER: *The forensic-expert-witness world is so widely populated with divas who perceive any person with half a brain as a threat to them. Cyril loves to encourage ideas, and he's not threatened by others people's competence. In fact, he loves it.*

I can't say that my business is a pleasant one. I'm always being challenged by somebody. But when those challenges are confrontational, they just intensify my emotional investment; I want to prevail all the more. If I didn't take things personally and was strictly in it for the money, I would have far fewer problems. But what I do means something to me, and to the people I serve.

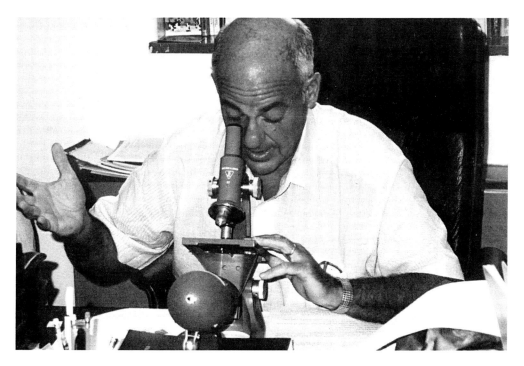

At work.

GERALDO RIVERA: *I'd bet on Cyril any time as a witness as opposed to any of the other first-tier forensic pathologists. He's really a legend in his field, however controversial. He's well regarded and dreaded if someone's opposing him.*

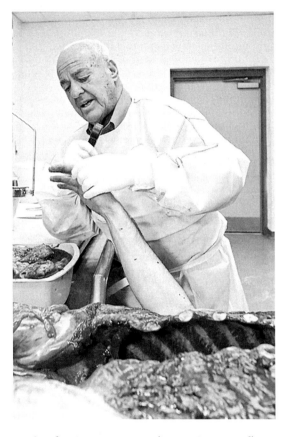

Conducting an autopsy (Renee Rosensteel).

I don't want to wave the flag of justice, but it hurts me greatly when there's a malpractice case, or a wrongful death suit of any kind, and I feel that the science is solid and the verdict goes against the victim and their family. Sometimes, I allow myself to become too emotionally invested, and I'm glad that I don't look at these things in some perfunctory fashion. Obviously, not every case has the same kind of emotionalism attached to it, and not every case is famous or controversial. And not every case is significant and important, in a broad sense. Every case, however, means something to somebody. It could be a Worker's Compensation claim, or the fate of a retired coal miner who's suffering from black lung. The case could mean everything to a person and his or her family. I never lose sight of that.

ALAN DERSHOWITZ: *Cyril will be talked about until the end of time because he has influenced so many people. When he started out, his profession was not highly regarded. Now, of course, the most popular shows on television are CSI dramas. Forensic science is "in" today. But in the days when he was first practicing, Cyril was a lone ranger and he, in many ways, created the profession, professionalized it, and made it into what it is today, which is central to the administration of justice. But there's another thing: Cyril has tremendous credibility. He is not a witness-for-hire. He's a witness for truth.*

Contributors

The following individuals were interviewed by Jeff Sewald for this book for the purpose of supporting my narrative and commentary, and elaborating on my story and my work. We wish to thank them all for their willingness to contribute to the portrait of me painted herein.

Gary Aguilar, M.D.—Ophthalmologist, researcher, and critic of the Warren Commission Report.

Stanley Albright—Jury member for my federal trial.

Honorable Ruggero Aldisert (now deceased)—Pittsburgh judge who was appointed to the U.S. Court of Appeals for the Third Circuit, and who served with distinction until age 94.

Ken Bacha—Westmoreland County Coroner. I have been conducting autopsies for that county for decades, for Ken and for his father, Leo Bacha, before him.

Dr. Michael Baden—Former Chief Medical Examiner of New York City and former Chief Forensic Pathologist for the New York State Police, now in private practice. Dr. Baden and I have worked on many cases together.

F. Lee Bailey, Esq.—Criminal defense attorney famous for defending, among many others, Albert DeSalvo ("The Boston Strangler"), Sam Sheppard, Patty Hearst, and O.J. Simpson.

Alec Baldwin—Famous stage, screen and television actor who played Dr. Julian Bailes in the film *Concussion*, which focused on pathologist Dr. Bennet Omalu (who worked for me) and the truth about brain damage in football players.

Harold Balk, Esq.—My son-in-law, married to my daughter, Dr. Ingrid Wecht.

Alvin Berkun—Rabbi, formerly of the Tree of Life Synagogue in Pittsburgh.

Bob Bible—Jury member for my federal trial.

Nicholas Cafardi, Esq.—Former Dean of the Duquesne University School of Law, and former U.S. Legal Attaché to the Vatican.

Ellis Cannon—Pittsburgh-area television and radio personality.

Dawn Cashmere—Jury member for my federal trial.

Stephen Catanzarite—Chairman of the Midland Innovation and Technology Charter School and managing director of the Lincoln Park Performing Arts Center.

Bob Del Greco, Esq.—Prominent criminal defense attorney in Pittsburgh.

Alan Dershowitz, Esq.—Distinguished Professor of Law at Harvard University (retired) and criminal defense attorney famous for defending, among others, Claus von Bülow, WikiLeaks founder Julian Assange, televangelist Jim Bakker, hotelier Leona Helmsley, and O.J. Simpson.

Joseph Dominick, R.N.—Chief Deputy Coroner under me before my federal trial began.

Donnie Eichar—Co-writer and co-producer of *Soaked in Bleach*, a documentary about the mysterious death of rock star Kurt Cobain.

Buck Favorini—Former head of the University of Pittsburgh Department of Theatre Arts.

Ronald Freeman (now deceased)—Former Commander of the Pittsburgh Police Homicide Division, with whom I worked on many murder cases when I was Allegheny County Coroner.

Sister Grace Ann Geibel, Ph.D. (now deceased)—Former President of Carlow University in Pittsburgh who established the forensic science and autopsy program at Carlow, and appointed me "Distinguished Professor of Pathology and Forensic Science."

Mark Geragos, Esq.—Top-level criminal defense attorney, famous for defending, among others, Michael Jackson and Scott Peterson.

Ken Gormley, Esq.—President of Duquesne University, home of the Cyril H. Wecht Institute of Forensic Science and Law.

Stuart Grodd—A close friend in New Haven, Connecticut, since my early teens.

Dr. Arthur Grossman—Optometrist (retired) and a close friend since my years at the University of Pittsburgh.

Dr. Sanjay Gupta—Neurosurgeon and TV medical reporter for CNN, and other media outlets.

Donald Guter, Esq.—Former Dean of the Duquesne University School of Law, Rear Admiral in the U.S. Navy (retired), and former President and Dean of the South Texas College of Law.

Jennifer Hammers, D.O.—Forensic pathologist and my assistant since July 2017.

Franco Harris—Former Pittsburgh Steelers running back and NFL Hall of Fame inductee.

Samuel Hazo—Retired University of Pittsburgh professor, renowned poet, and a good friend.

Heather Heidelbaugh, Esq.—Pittsburgh trial lawyer for Leech, Tishman, Fuscaldo and Lampl.

Alan Jerry Johnson, Esq.—Former U.S. Attorney for the Western District of Pennsylvania, and a good friend.

Kimberly Jones—Jury member for my federal trial.

Dawna Kaufmann—Investigative journalist, reporter and television commentator who has co-authored three books with me.

Louis "Hop" Kendrick—African American community leader in Pittsburgh and a personal friend since my days at Fifth Avenue High School.

Andrew Kreig, Esq.—Attorney and investigative journalist.

Peter Landesman—Producer, writer and director of the film *Concussion*, about pathologist Dr. Bennet Omalu (who worked for me) and the truth about brain damage in football players.

Mark Lane, Esq. (now deceased)—Prominent criminal defense attorney and one of the early critics of the Warren Commission Report, who wrote *Rush to Judgment*, about the JFK assassination.

Dr. Henry Lee—Internationally renowned criminalist and founder of the Henry C. Lee Institute at the University of New Haven, Connecticut.

Kerry Lewis—Criminal defense attorney in Pittsburgh who represented the family of Charles Dixon in the case that was a precipitating factor for the federal corruption case that was filed against me.

Joseph Mancuso—My longtime autopsy assistant at the Allegheny County Coroner's Office and now my private autopsy technician and prosector.

Dr. Joseph Maroon—Vice Chairman of the Department of Neurological Surgery at the University of Pittsburgh Medical Center (UPMC) and Heindl Scholar in Neuroscience. One of America's finest neurosurgeons, Joe is also the team neurosurgeon for the Pittsburgh Steelers football team.

Sophie Masloff (now deceased)—Former Mayor of the City of Pittsburgh, and a strong supporter.

Kathy McCabe—Former Allegheny County Coroner's Office secretary when I was at the helm.

Jerry McDevitt, Esq.—Prominent criminal defense attorney and senior partner at K&L Gates, Pittsburgh, who was the lead defense attorney for my federal corruption trial.

John McIntire—Pittsburgh television and radio personality on whose programs and in whose theatrical shows I have appeared many times.

Chris Moore—Pittsburgh television and radio host, and commentator.

Charles M. Morrison—Trooper First Class with the Pennsylvania State Police, who has worked as a forensic technician with me on a variety of cases.

Patrick Nightingale, Esq.—A former prosecutor and practicing criminal defense attorney, and an advocate of marijuana legalization, who used my expertise and experience about the issue to advance the cause.

Dr. Thomas Noguchi—Prominent forensic pathologist, former Chief Medical Examiner of Los Angeles County, who presided over the cases of Charles Manson, Marilyn Monroe, Robert F. Kennedy, Natalie Wood, among many others.

Tony Norman—Columnist for the *Pittsburgh Post-Gazette.*

Honorable John Peck, Esq.—Longtime District Attorney of Westmoreland County, for whom I have testified many times in homicide trials.

John Rago, Esq.—Professor at the Duquesne University School of Law School who played a key role in helping to establish the Cyril H. Wecht Institute of Forensic Science and Law there.

Katherine Ramsland—Forensic psychologist, true-crime author of more than 60 books, and Professor and Associate Provost at DeSales University in Center Valley, Pennsylvania.

Geraldo Rivera—Well-known television personality and TV host on whose shows I have appeared many times.

William Robinson—African American community leader in Pittsburgh, former Pennsylvania State Representative and member of Allegheny County Council, and a political supporter of mine.

Jim Roddey—Prominent businessman and community leader who defeated me in the Allegheny County Executive election in 1999, and now a personal friend.

Leon Rozin, M.D.—Forensic pathologist from Russia and Israel whom I hired at the Allegheny County Coroner's Office in the 1990s.

Mark Rush, Esq.—Attorney for the firm of K&L Gates, Pittsburgh, and co-counsel, with Jerry McDevitt, for my federal corruption trial.

June Schulberg, Esq. (now deceased)—Preeminent family law attorney, former Chief Deputy Coroner of Allegheny County and, previously, my personal secretary.

Mark Schwartz, Esq.—Attorney who shepherded the case of Robert Wideman, helping him to achieve his release from prison after serving more than 40 years.

L. Kathleen Sekula, Ph.D.—Professor of Nursing at Duquesne University who has been instrumental in establishing the strong collaboration between the university's School of Nursing and the Cyril H. Wecht Institute of Forensic Science and Law.

Susan Shanaman—Solicitor and Government Affairs Representative for the Pennsylvania State Coroners' Association.

Honorable Josh Shapiro, Esq.—Pennsylvania Attorney General, whom I encouraged to run for the office in 2016.

Sam Shapiro—One of my oldest and closest friends, and my fraternity brother at the University of Pittsburgh. I was best man at his wedding.

Francis Shine (now deceased)—One of my best friends at Fifth Avenue High School.

Bev Smith—Pittsburgh radio personality for many years and an active African American community leader.

Richard A. Sprague, Esq.—A prominent trial attorney and, for many years, Chief Prosecutor in the Philadelphia District Attorney's Office. Dick was appointed Chief Counsel for the U.S. House of Representatives Select Committee on Assassinations in 1977.

Joy Starzl—Widow of famed transplant surgeon Dr. Thomas Starzl, and a friend.

Ben Statler—Co-producer, co-writer and director of *Soaked in Bleach*, a documentary about the mysterious death of rock star Kurt Cobain, in which I am featured.

Oliver Stone—Oscar-winning writer and director with whom I consulted on his film *JFK*, and again on a new documentary about the JFK assassination.

Robert Tanenbaum, Esq.—Longtime head of the Manhattan District Attorney's Homicide Division who served as Deputy Chief Counsel for the House of Representatives Select Committee on Assassinations in 1977.

Bruce Thomas—Jury member for my federal trial.

Josiah Thompson, Ph.D.—Wrote the book *Six Seconds in Dallas* and invited me, in December of 1966, to study the Zapruder film at *Life* magazine headquarters in New York City.

Richard Thornburgh—Former U.S. Attorney for the Western District of Pennsylvania, Governor of Pennsylvania and, ultimately, U.S. Attorney General, who helped me to develop the defense for my federal corruption trial.

Sala Udin—African American community leader and former member of Pittsburgh City Council.

Tim Uhrich, Esq.—A Pittsburgh attorney who was a staff member when I ran for public office, and who served as Solicitor when I ran the Allegheny County Coroner's Office from 1996 to 2006.

Vic Walczak—Legal Director of the American Civil Liberties Union of Pennsylvania.

Ben Wecht—My youngest son and, since 2003, Director of the Cyril H. Wecht Institute of Forensic Science and Law at Duquesne University.

Daniel Wecht, M.D.—My middle son and prominent neurosurgeon at the University of Pittsburgh Medical Center (UPMC).

Honorable David Wecht—My oldest son and a Pennsylvania Supreme Court Justice.

Ingrid Wecht, M.D.—My only daughter and an obstetrician-gynecologist in private practice at West Penn Hospital in Pittsburgh.

Sigrid Wecht, Esq.—My wife of nearly 60 years and my strongest and most important supporter, who works full-time as the executive administrator in my private office.

Michael Welner, M.D.—Originally from Pittsburgh, now a prominent forensic psychiatrist in New York City.

John Edgar Wideman—Rhodes Scholar and award-winning author, originally from Pittsburgh.

Eileen Young—A loyal and strong supporter, longtime secretary at the Allegheny County Coroner's Office, and former chief secretary in my private office.

The Authors in Brief

Dr. Cyril H. Wecht, M.D., J.D., is a forensic pathologist, attorney and medical-legal consultant. He is certified by the American Board of Pathology in anatomic, clinical and forensic pathology, the American Board of Legal Medicine, and the American Board of Disaster Medicine. He is also a Fellow of the College of American Pathologists and the American Society of Clinical Pathologists. Dr. Wecht has served as President of the American College of Legal Medicine and the American Academy of Forensic Sciences, and was Chairman of the Board of Trustees of the American Board of Legal Medicine and the American College of Legal Medicine Foundation. For 19 years, he served as the elected Coroner of Pennsylvania's Allegheny County. The building in which he once worked is now named for him. He continues to testify in criminal and civil trials around the world, as both a prosecution and defense expert witness.

Jeff Sewald is an award-winning writer and filmmaker who specializes in defining the cultural significance of people, places, things and events. Through the years, his work has brought him in contact with a host of luminaries including American historian and author David McCullough, television news anchor Tom Brokaw, film director Sidney Lumet, the NFL's Mike Ditka, and rock music legend Lou Reed. In addition to his newspaper and magazine work, Mr. Sewald's films include *Gridiron & Steel*, a documentary focusing on the spiritual relationship that exists between the sport of football and the people of southwestern Pennsylvania; *Peter Matthiessen: No Boundaries*, about the legendary author and environmentalist; and *We Knew What We Had: The Greatest Jazz Story Never Told* which chronicles the history and significance of jazz music in his hometown of Pittsburgh.

Other Books
by Cyril Wecht

Cyril Wecht is the author or co-author of 45 professional books for doctors and lawyers, and the five-volume set *Forensic Sciences*, which was published in 1982 and is still in print, supported by semiannual supplements. He has also published the following popular books:

Cause of Death: The Shocking True Stories Behind the Headlines—A Forensic Expert Speaks Out on JFK, RFK, Elvis, Chappaquiddick, and Other Controversial Cases (with Mark Curriden and Benjamin Wecht)

Final Exams: True Crime Cases from Cyril Wecht (with Dawna Kaufmann)

From Crime Scene to Courtroom (with Dawna Kaufmann)

Grave Secrets: A Leading Forensic Expert Reveals the Startling Truth about O.J. Simpson, David Koresh, Vincent Foster, and Other Sensational Cases (with Mark Curriden and Benjamin Wecht)

Mortal Evidence: The Forensics Behind Nine Shocking Cases (with Greg Saitz and Mark Curriden)

A Question of Murder: Compelling Cases from a Famed Forensic Pathologist including Anna Nicole Smith, Daniel Smith, and More (with Dawna Kaufmann)

Tales from the Morgue: Forensic Answers to Nine Famous Cases including Scott Peterson and Chandra Levy (with Mark Curriden and Angela Powell)

Who Killed JonBenét Ramsey? A Leading Forensic Expert Uncovers the Shocking Facts (with Charles Bosworth)

Index

Index